JONNO PROUDFOOT

THE ★ REAL MEAL REVOLUTION 2.0

REAL MEAL REVOLUTION

"My wife just handed me *The Real Meal Revolution* and told me that we were going on this diet. I've lost a total of 9½ stone. I no longer struggle to get up the stairs."
– **SKIP, 60**

"My Real Meal Revolution began when I was dreading wearing a swimsuit on holiday. I was insecure, I always felt tired and my body ached. Since I started the diet I feel so much better and have lost about a stone. It is the first time in a long time that I feel so great."
– Anne-Marie, 37

"I have tried many diets, but I never stuck with any of them. Again and again I would buy a new wardrobe. I didn't get the Real Meal Revolution principle at first, but falling off the wagon taught me that this is not a diet – it is a lifestyle. I've lost over 2 stone and I'm at my optimum weight."
– SAMANTHA, 32

★ ★ ★ ★ ★

"I was about to get bariatric surgery, but decided to try one more healthy weight-loss programme before going under the knife. Four years later I've lost 11½ stone through the Real Meal Revolution. I feel like I've been given a second chance. It saved my life."
– **BRIAN, 49** (@BrianBerkmanZa)

"I am a personal trainer and an ex-professional dancer. I have always been relatively healthy, and I have loosely followed diets like Atkins, Protein Power Life Plan, South Beach Diet, etc. I now refer many of my clients to the Real Meal Revolution: it's changed my life by waking me up to be more informed on healthy lifestyle trends."

– MALCOLM, 41

"I began my RMR diet journey at 11 stone 11lb, and I now weigh 9 stone 8lb. My weight loss may not be massive by others' standards, but the impact on my body, self-esteem and the way I view myself is immense. I feel reborn, young and have a zest for life!"

– FAIEZA, 52

"I have an active lifestyle. I run and do yoga and Pilates. The RMR diet helps me keep up with my active lifestyle and avoid feeling hungry or tired through my workouts."

– STACI, 45

"I've lost 7½ stone. I cannot express how well I feel. The health benefits that have come with the weight loss have been liberating – no more heartburn, no more snoring, no knee pain, no bloating and no slugishness. I feel absolutely great!"

– Nina, 42

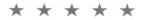

JONNO PROUDFOOT is a food expert, entrepreneur and adventurer, and the driving force behind the Real Meal Revolution (RMR) brand. He conceptualised and co-authored the bestselling *Real Meal Revolution* and *Raising Superheroes*, both of which have been published internationally.

REAL MEAL REVOLUTION is the fastest-growing diet company in South Africa, specialising in online and face-to-face weight-loss and healthy-eating support.

Key book contributors include:

BRIDGET SURTEES: registered dietitian with experience in London, Sydney and Cape Town; co-author of *Raising Superheroes*;

KAREN HARTZENBERG: medical doctor specialising in LCHF eating; believes in real data and randomised control trials;

GUSS DAVEY: computer scientist and numbers specialist; responsible for crunching much of the big data in these pages;

LEAINE BREBNER: RMR's head of content; collator of feedback from thousands of clients, experts, books, journals, talks and more;

ROB HICHENS: qualified sports scientist and manager of RMR's elite diet coaches; the practical hand;

ROB WORTHINGTON-SMITH: experienced popular science writer; helped make the difficult stuff easy to understand.

First published in South Africa in 2017 by Mercury, an imprint of Burnet Media, in collaboration with Real Meal Revolution

•

First published in Great Britain in 2017 by Robinson

•

1 3 5 7 9 10 8 6 4 2

•

•

IMPORTANT NOTE
The recommendations in this book are solely intended as education
and information and should not be taken as medical advice.

•

A CIP catalogue record for this book
is available from the British Library.

•

ISBN: 978-1-40871-019-7

•

Typeset in Melior 10pt on 15pt
Printed and bound in Great Britain by Clays Ltd, St Ives plc

•

Papers used by Robinson are from well-managed forests and other responsible sources.

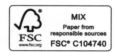

Robinson
An imprint of
Little, Brown Book Group
Carmelite House
50 Victoria Embankment
London EC4Y 0DZ

•

An Hachette UK Company
www.hachette.co.uk
www.littlebrown.co.uk

To the Real Meal Revolution team,
who work their butts off every day
to help change people's lives

CONTENTS

PART 1:
THE OVERVIEW

PART 2:
REAL MEAL 2.0:
THE DIET, THE LIFESTYLE

PART 3:
HACKS, FAQS & OTHER RESOURCES

PART 4:
RECIPES & MEAL PLANS

PART 1
OVERVIEW

1.1 INTRODUCTION
BY JONNO PROUDFOOT

The most important dietary revelation of the last 40 years is this: fat is not the enemy, whereas carbohydrates may well be – and, in particular, we need to be wary of sugar.

I call it a revelation but this knowledge is something we humans once knew and subsequently lost. For thousands of years our ancestors instinctively ate according to this rule, and later the doctors and early dietitians of the 19th and 20th century were intimately aware of it. We abruptly abandoned the rule in the late 1970s so the importance of its "rediscovery" in the early 21st century must be given context: the critical point is that we've largely been applying the opposite principle for the last four decades. (There's a fuller explanation of how this happened from p30.)

In recent decades we have been fuelling ourselves primarily with carbohydrates, and in doing so we have brought a blight on human health and happiness. An epidemic of obesity and dietary-related illness has swept the world, originating in the United States and advancing wherever fast-food retailers and Western-style shopping malls can be found. Should it continue unchecked, things will unfortunately get worse; our collective health will deteriorate and the economic effects will be profound.

This book, and the Real Meal Revolution in general, is underscored by the notion that we need to embrace fat and be wary of carbohydrates in our diet. Objective science says as much and the point has largely been proven.

But it's time for the next step in the process. This simple, broad (but critical) revelation has been heard by many around the world; now we have the evidence and feedback to offer a more nuanced, targeted approach to the sometimes complex matter of losing weight and being healthy.

Welcome to the evolution of *The Real Meal Revolution*.

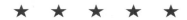

I am not a veteran journalist trained in applied physics who has systematically reviewed a century of scientific data to debunk the diet-heart hypothesis (Gary Taubes); nor am I a kidney specialist who observed the links between his patients' insulin problems and obesity in his daily practice (Jason Fung); nor am I even scientifically trained like most of the key figures leading the global low-carb high-fat (LCHF) movement. I am a chef with an accounting degree and a sense of adventure, and I can thank my girlfriend (now wife) Kate for opening my eyes to the potential of LCHF and steering me, inadvertently or otherwise, into a career based around this way of eating. Let me outline my journey briefly as a way of explaining the rationale and intentions of this book.

In 2010, after finishing a half Iron Man in East London, in South Africa, I made a gentleman's agreement with my training partner, Thane Williams, to complete a physical challenge that we hoped would leave a mark on the history books. We wanted to achieve a world first and we eventually settled on swimming the Mozambique Channel, the body of water that separates the continent of Africa from the island of Madagascar. The channel is

260 miles (420km) at its narrowest point so it was an ambitious goal: it would take us four years of planning and fund-raising before we could achieve it, and my life would change irreversibly in that time.

With my business hat on, I thought it would make sense to develop a product of some sort to earn money in annuity for our chosen charity, Miles for Smiles, rather than actively soliciting donations at talks and events, a time-consuming and ongoing process. So I hit upon the idea of creating a cookbook that would focus on the food Thane and I ate while training for our epic mission. I just needed an angle for the cookbook...

Coincidentally, 2010 also saw the start of another epic mission, though this one would have more far-reaching results. In this case, 2010 was the year that Professor Tim Noakes turned his back on the carbohydrate-based diet he'd been following (and prescribing) since his days as a young medical professional in the late 1970s. Despite rigorously following the recommended low-fat guidelines, Prof Noakes found he had developed the type-2 diabetes that ran in his family. As a result, he concluded that the experts who advocated the guidelines must be mistaken and he returned to the fat-based whole foods of his younger days, a "Damascene conversion" that saw him shed 3 stone with relative ease and significantly improve his general health and running times for the first time in a decade.

To that point, Prof Noakes was renowned publicly as South Africa's top sports scientist: one of the country's esteemed A1-rated academics, an expert on endurance running, among other things, and an advocate of "challenging beliefs" (as the title of his biography published in 2011 would attest). By early 2013, he was making a new name for himself in radio interviews and online articles as a proponent of low-carb eating. Weight gain and loss were closely related to something called insulin resistance, he explained, and the long-term result of our modern, refined, carb-laden diet was obesity and ill health. In closely following the latest dietary science and monitoring the performances of numerous top local athletes who'd turned to LCHF eating, he felt more and more strongly that the wisdom of crowds would trump the increasingly questioned authority of the nutritional establishment. Word of "the Noakes diet" spread.

It was at this point that Kate thought she would give the diet a go, and over the course of six months she also lost, as the Prof had done before her, 3 stone. The effects were dramatic and the logic compelling. What's more, the food was delicious, even decadent. I realised I had found the angle for my cookbook, and that Thane and I would train for our swim to Madagascar powered by butter, bacon and broccoli.

The second half of 2013 was a surreal blur of action and creativity, inspired by the news that Prof Noakes was keen to be involved in my project, along with chef-adventurer David Grier and nutritionist Sally-Ann Creed. We met in July to start the process of turning my framework into a book to change the world, and it took just 63 days from that point until we sent our book to print, a ludicrously short time-frame to write, shoot, edit and lay out a full-colour science-cum-recipe book (we wanted the book out for Christmas). In the end, the creative energy was right and, as it turned out, we'd nailed the dietary zeitgeist.

The Real Meal Revolution went straight to number one on the South African charts and for the first year we lost top spot briefly only when we ran out of stock. In a year we sold 150,000 copies, a phenomenal feat in our small reading market, and by late 2016 we'd almost doubled that figure. In 2015 the book was published internationally by Little, Brown of London, one of the world's premier publishers. In 2016 they also published our follow-up title on nutrition for children, *Raising Superheroes* (as *Super Food For Superchildren*), another South African bestseller.

Even today I look at these facts and figures with a mixture of astonishment and incredible gratitude for the success of *The Real Meal Revolution* – and also with the understanding that there is a healthy element of luck involved. All first-time authors will tell you they want nothing short of a bestseller, but anyone who's been in the publishing industry for longer than five minutes knows just how slim the chances of success are. We achieved it because South Africans didn't just want a book on low-carb eating; they *needed* it. Since the release of *The Real Meal Revolution*, similar LCHF recipe books have also sold well; we just happened to get there first and we had the influence of Professor Tim Noakes to publicise our book.

2014 turned out to be an incredible year. The book didn't stop selling, Thane and I swam to Madagascar, Kate and I got married, and I effectively started a new business based on the power of the Real Meal Revolution (RMR) brand. After taking advice and considering my options, I decided to put together an online course on the RealMealRevolution.com website that I'd registered the previous year, which at that point simply hosted miscellaneous bits and pieces to do with the book. I presented my plans to a potential tech-company partner and the analytics convinced them; turns out my no-frills website was already generating enormous amounts of traffic.

Some people call the type of LCHF eating we were advocating "Banting", after the person who first made it popular (see p22). In time, we came to think of it as a lifestyle – a Real Meal Revolution – and in this book you'll find it referred to as the RMR diet. But in October 2014 we launched a state-of-the-art online "Banting course", which included various media, plans, recipes and tools. We had developed one noteworthy piece of software in particular, a meal tracker to track macronutrient ratios and carb counts of various meals. We thought it was pretty cool and hoped it would make the experience more user-friendly – it did, and as it turns out it became a brilliant and valuable source of data for us.

The incredible public response to *The Real Meal Revolution* has continued to drive our business. At the time of writing, we have accumulated data from more than 120,000 free trials run through our site. Even more useful information has come from the 6,000 users who've signed up to our courses and, of these, the more than 1,200 who have tracked their meals every day for more than 100 days and tracked their weight more than 30 times. Our courses were not designed as scientific studies, but the practical data and feedback have been eye-opening.

Our searchable chat forum has been a similarly valuable resource, allowing us to identify and track common questions and problems. In time, we find the answers and solutions, often with the help and further feedback of those on the forums.

Beyond the critical user feedback, the success of *The Real Meal Revolution* and our relationship with Prof Noakes plugged the RMR business into the global network of LCHF experts. We interact mostly online (where the democratisation of nutritional information is most effective) but also in person. In February 2015 Karen Thomson and Prof Noakes co-hosted the world's first low-carb high-fat convention (officially the Old Mutual Health

Convention), which saw 16 renowned LCHF specialists come together in Cape Town. RMR filmed and produced the entire convention online. It was a remarkable event that helped us identify critical nodes of knowledge around the world. Many of those in attendance, such as Gary Taubes and Jason Fung, mentioned earlier, are represented in *The Experts* from p175.

And so, with what is effectively an enormous resource library of clearly quantified data, real-life stories and expert advice, the platform has been set to refine the Real Meal Revolution approach and take it into the future. This book is the result.

Among the various life lessons the tremendous sales of *The Real Meal Revolution* have taught me, I discovered two interesting aspects to this thing called success. One, it can be difficult and demanding. And two, it is fleeting and sometimes even intangible.

The difficult side came most obviously with our exposure to the extreme polarities of the low-carb versus low-fat debate, and the ensuing public controversy. As Prof Noakes used his prominence in the public eye to promote the book, the critical backlash he and we received from those professionals who had invested their careers and beliefs in low-fat eating was often jaw-dropping. To this day the backlash continues, despite the ever increasing weight of widely accepted science in our favour. (Though Prof Noakes and RMR operate independently, for the most part, we are often seen to be affiliated and take flak for each other's work.)

It was important to get my head around this defensive human response to protect one's territory because these clashes of the scientific and medical heavyweights frequently left us mere mortals wondering where to turn. Many of the major objections on both sides of the debate used the same arguments and often even the same language: the other side was always "cherry-picking" data in its attempts to "demonise" carbs/fats.

Amid the chaos and controversy, I noticed how those potentially interested in LCHF eating were frequently left with unanswered questions:

Isn't all that fat going to kill me?

How do I know if I'm insulin resistant?

How can changing what I eat affect my health?

Why should I eat differently if I'm already on medication to manage my condition?

Should I worry about my cholesterol?

How many cappuccinos can I drink in a day?

Who do I believe?

The science was confusing and often overwhelming. Many readers simply cooked from the recipes and winged the actual diet.

It became clear that we had provided the broad strokes to a dietary revolution but that there were gaps to be filled and grey areas to be coloured. Our original success in the book format demanded we be more accurate and clear as we moved ahead. We needed to look beyond the single revelatory truth; yes, carbs are generally bad and fat is generally good, but the rule affects people to different degrees. Moreover, diet is just one piece of the sometimes complex weight-health pie; there are various other factors, such as stress, sleep and exercise, that must be acknowledged and catered for.

The fleeting nature of success was evident in the amount of work still to be done. Whenever I received a book sales report or heard a random person discussing the diet and the Real Meal Revolution in public, I was amazed at what we'd achieved, and yet the real success now lay in spreading the message even further. More than two-billion humans, nearly a third of the world population, are considered overweight or obese. *Real* success would come in reaching not hundreds of thousands of people, but hundreds of millions of people. In February 2015 I set our company a BHAG (that's short for Big Hairy Audacious Goal, as Jim Collins followers will know): in ten years, by 2025, the Real Meal Revolution will have changed 100-million lives.

Now *that* will be success.

In the meantime, the tangibility of success strikes home in the stories of the individuals whose lives have been utterly, profoundly changed for the better by following the RMR diet.

The most successful RMR dieter in terms of sheer weight loss, AJ, lost a mind-blowing 21½ stone over the course of two years from a peak weight of over 44 stone. Now 32, he has started running half marathons and mountain biking and his goal is to complete an Iron Man in 2017.

More recently a husband-and-wife team, Nina and Rowan, lost a combined 13½ stone between them, having once believed they would "die fat". The many maladies they shared – snoring, knee pain, bloating, heartburn – are a thing of the past.

The many extreme weight-loss stories obviously stand out but the real success is measured in more than just pounds and inches. Whether it's seeing the results of a weight-loss intervention project in a disadvantaged community, working with people who've been so positively affected by their experiences that they've decided to become professional RMR diet coaches, or simply talking to someone I've just met at a party who's lost a bit of weight and is feeling much better for it, a common theme is one of being uplifted and empowered.

These are the types of people we have interacted with on a daily basis over the last three years. For all the scientific debate I've followed and the data I've seen tortured in that time (to whatever agenda), it's these real people losing weight and becoming healthier in the real world that show the way ahead. We now have the data, experience and interconnected global knowledge to help recreate success stories like these with ever more regularity by allowing people to understand their bodies' specific needs.

Looking back, I like to think of the original *Real Meal Revolution* as a call to turn around the collective ship of human wellbeing. Sailing towards mass obesity and ill health, powered by carbs, we needed a 180-degree course change – and the revelation that fat is our friend was that change. Now it's time to work out the bearing of your own individual vessel, and Real Meal 2.0 has been put together to allow you to do just that.

I hope this book puts you on the right course to a healthy life.

1.2 A GUIDE TO THE GUIDE

Now, let's get into the best way to use this book.

Our most important piece of advice upfront: please don't be tempted to skip ahead to the Diet in Part II and start today.

Almost all diets work initially – and almost all diets fail eventually. One of the key principles we've learnt at RMR is the importance of preparation and observation in achieving sustainable results: you will greatly increase your chances for long-term success if you don't jump ahead. This will also give us the opportunity to convey the importance of the concept of the RMR diet as a lifestyle, rather than as just a diet.

For now, here are some key questions to start the journey.

WHAT WAS BANTING?

In the original *Real Meal Revolution*, we effectively reinvigorated the old dietary term "Banting" as a synonym for LCHF (low-carb high-fat). Originating from William Banting, the man who popularised low-carb eating in the UK in the second half of the 19th century, we figured a catchy name would be more powerful than a boring abbreviation, and would allow us the room to put our own spin on LCHF eating.

To Bant was thus to limit your carbohydrate intake, with the aim of switching your body's metabolism from being primarily carb-fuelled to being primarily fat-fuelled. A severe carb restriction would stop you storing energy as body fat and encourage you to use your stored energy (body fat) to run your body's functions. Once you had lost sufficient body fat, you would use dietary fat (rather than dietary carbs) to run your body's functions and sustain the weight loss and health benefits in the long term.

(Note that Banting was never a licence to gorge on fat without limit, a misconception that occasionally arose after the release of *The Real Meal Revolution*. See p85 for more on this.)

Beyond this, our first version of Banting promoted the consumption of "real" ingredients and rejected the refined and adulterated foods that have come to dominate modern consumer living. In the misguided age of low-fat eating, with sugar and artificial flavourants pervading so much of what we eat, Banting was a fundamental step in curbing the ever climbing rates of obesity around the world.

WHAT IS REAL MEAL 2.0?

Three years after our first book, Real Meal 2.0 is the evolution of the revolution. In essence, we see it as eating real food to regenerate your health, one element of which is carbohydrate restriction. We call it the RMR diet here, but you might also come across references to "Banting".

We see Real Meal 2.0 as the finessing of a specific approach to diet that now incorporates a broader, holistic approach to both diet and living in a way that will help you to be healthier. Managing your weight with what you eat is still essential to the plan, but now we're giving emphasis to the concept of lifestyle – because losing weight and being healthy isn't just about eating correctly; it's about recognising all the variables that affect the way your body runs and getting them to work together in harmony. It's about eating and living well, enjoying your food and how you spend your time, getting the most out of life and being healthy in a sustainable way.

It's about getting from overweight and underperforming – and even chronically ill in many instances – to energised, happy and healthy. It is, in short, about getting to Awesome.

WHAT IS INSULIN RESISTANCE AND WHY ARE HORMONES SO IMPORTANT?

The basis for the RMR diet lies in a hormonal explanation for why we get fat, with insulin being the most important and commonly discussed culprit. Among other things, insulin regulates the amount of glucose in the blood, telling fat cells when to take in glucose and convert it to fat. The often-discussed "insulin resistance" is a failure of the body to respond as it should when insulin is released, in which case ever-increasing amounts of insulin are released. A vicious cycle of fat accumulation and increased insulin levels ensues, of which a pervasive side effect is chronic inflammation. An important aspect of the RMR diet is working out how insulin resistant you are (see p167).

The RMR diet, along with other LCHF ways of eating, seeks to limit the amount of insulin in the system by reducing the intake of glucose and allowing the body to convert its already stored glucose, in fat cells, into energy. In so doing, the fat cells are burnt off. This is done most obviously by regulating what you eat, but also by keeping in check the levels of other important hormones that affect insulin, such as cortisol and adrenaline. A key aspect of making this switch is a naturally reduced appetite, which returns the body to a virtuous health/eating cycle.

Thus the RMR diet looks to keep our hormones regulated in a healthy way, focusing both directly and indirectly on insulin by considering other important hormones too.

WHO SHOULD MAKE THE SWITCH?

We believe that most people would benefit from the RMR to diet to a greater or lesser degree. Certainly we strongly recommend it for anyone who is considerably overweight, diabetic or pre-diabetic and/or highly insulin resistant; the results we've seen with such people have been nothing short of incredible.

Though not everyone will need to severely restrict their carb intake as per the Transformation phase of Real Meal 2.0 (see p119), everyone will benefit from eating the real foods and healthy fats we advocate. We advise Preservation (see p124) for almost anyone, even if you're not looking to lose weight, both for direct health implications today and to pre-empt future problems.

The guiding idea behind *Raising Superheroes*, our book on children's and family nutrition, was based on this latter idea. We wanted to set up the next generation for good health rather than trying to fix problems down the line, and in so doing we advocated what we now consider to be the mildest form of the RMR diet: avoiding sugar and refined carbs where possible, and eating real food. This concept applies to almost anyone who is currently healthy and wishes to stay that way for the rest of their life.

Moreover, Real Meal 2.0 layers further lifestyle benefits on top of the original benefits of *The Real Meal Revolution* approach to eating, effectively giving you more opportunities to be healthy.

Remember, though: it is advisable to consult your doctor before embarking on any diet or weight-loss plan.

WHAT ARE THE BENEFITS OF THE RMR DIET?

There are huge health benefits across so many facets of our lives when we eat well. For a list of the diseases, conditions and maladies known to be affected by diet, see p47 (prepare to have your mind blown). Moreover, being healthy and confident in your body is liberating; it literally makes you happier.

WHAT ARE THE REAL MEAL REVOLUTION BELIEFS?

We believe in healthy fats, avoiding adulterated processed food, particularly refined carbohydrates, and taking a broad and holistic view to food, drink and life in general.

We believe in the miracles of modern science and medicine but disagree with the unnecessary chronic medication of vast swathes of the global population today – especially when eating and living well is a real alternative to fixing so many long-term problems, from critical health issues such as diabetes and liver disease to mental focus and energy levels to simply enjoying life and improving your golf game.

We believe each individual needs a customised approach to losing weight and feeling good, which they must work out for themselves, and that people are empowered and liberated by taking ownership of their health and wellbeing.

We are wary of conspiracy theorists and vitamin pedlars but we are equally wary of the motives that drive the Big Pharma and Big Food industries, and are sceptical of their data and particularly the dietary advice they feed us.

A NOTE ON THE SCIENCE, RESOURCES AND REFERENCING

The internet, for all its faults, allows us access to information that we only dreamt of seeing in the 1970s and '80s, when the guidelines that came to influence the modern Western diet were implemented (see p30). One of the resulting problems, however, is that we are now swimming in facts and figures, and it can be difficult for readers (or online users) to make head or tail of it all.

When it comes to contested aspects of the science or specific medical queries, we always recommend that readers educate themselves as much as possible: read the books and online articles on the topics that affect you personally and drill down to the actual studies that are referenced. And, of course, consult your doctor if you have a specific medical query.

In our previous books, *The Real Meal Revolution* and *Raising Superheroes*, we provided detailed science with meticulous referencing. In this book, however, we have chosen to pare down the science to make it clear, straightforward and easier to understand. Only when we feel it's absolutely necessary will we get a little technical.

This approach inevitably sees a trade-off between ease of understanding and rigorous academic scrutiny; we acknowledge this and the dangers inherent, though we think the end goal is worth it. To offset it where possible, we recommend further reading for particular sections as they arise. We have included an author resources section, *The Experts*, from p175 to acknowledge the experts whose work has helped us to refine our approach to the LCHF lifestyle; and we have included a detailed bibliography for the book at RealMealRevolution.com.

1.3 THE SCIENCE OF REAL MEAL 2.0

"The food you eat can either be the safest and most powerful form of medicine or the slowest form of poison."

– Aseem Malhotra, cardiologist and anti-sugar advocate

The Real Meal Revolution sparked a mass change in eating across the length and breadth of South Africa for a simple reason: it works. In short, people lost weight – a ton of it.

Those who have read *The Real Meal Revolution*, *Raising Superheroes* or other modern LCHF publications should have a good understanding of the science behind why this is so, as well as the history of how we came to get it so wrong in the first place.

For our purposes here, we need only a short recap of this before moving on to overviews of the four major mechanisms behind modern human obesity and ill health: insulin resistance, gut problems, gluten sensitivity and chronic inflammation. All have seen notable research progress since the publication of *The Real Meal Revolution*, and Real Meal 2.0 has been specifically refined to counter them all.

1.3.1 FAILED STATE v IDEAL STATE

The guiding hypothesis behind the RMR diet is that humans have two primary food-processing states: a slower metabolic fat-storage state and a faster metabolic fat-burning state.

The fat-storage state is initiated when you eat significantly more carbs than fat in your diet. Carbs stimulate insulin to keep blood-sugar levels in a safe range. But there are four other key roles insulin plays to keep you in fat-storage mode: it slows down your metabolism (so you burn less fuel and feel lethargic and less inclined to exercise); it sends messages to the appestat in your brain to continue feeling hungry, encouraging you to eat more, even if you've had enough; it passes the excess energy to the liver, which stores it in your tummy roll; and it blocks your metabolism from accessing these fat stores for energy, even when you feel hungry.

In time, the fat-storage state leads to a steady increase in weight and a converse decline in health and wellbeing. But in the fat-burning state, in which we primarily burn fats for energy, we remain lean, healthy and energised.

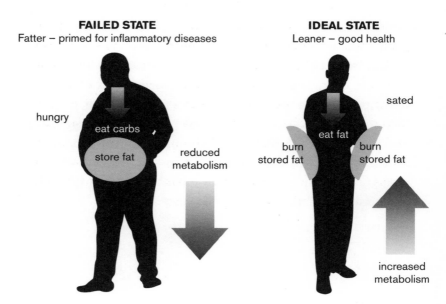

FAILED STATE
Fatter – primed for inflammatory diseases

hungry

eat carbs

store fat

reduced metabolism

IDEAL STATE
Leaner – good health

sated

eat fat

burn stored fat   burn stored fat

increased metabolism

THE OBESITY EPIDEMIC

How is it that so many of us are stuck in the fat-storage state these days, rather than the "natural" healthy fat-burning state? Here's the lowdown.

Once upon a time we were hunters and gatherers who lived off the land. Life was more brutish and shorter back in pre-civilised times, but we were optimally fit, as we need to be to survive, living primarily in a fat-burning state. With the advent of human settlement and agriculture came a steadier supply of carbohydrates, with more opportunity for us to get into the fat-storage state. The problems of regularly eating grains and other complex carbohydrates have been exacerbated over the millennia as we've industrialised, with increasing amounts of sugar and refined and processed foods in our diet. The health paradox of the modern age is upon us: despite our technological progression, we're less fit than we were and we're chronically unhealthy.

Several excellent books have now been written about how exactly this occurred – see our recommended reading on p35. Suffice to say that it was a complex (and often fascinating) combination of human politics and personality at its worst that saw the introduction of eating guidelines in the United States in 1977 recommending extremely high levels of carbohydrate consumption. These were the inaugural United States Dietary Goals for Americans (USDGA), and the year was a momentous tipping point in the history of collective human health.

The result has seen an American-led global obesity epidemic emerge over the last four decades, spreading from country to country and bringing with it a rise in a host of disastrous chronic diseases. According to the World Health Organization, global obesity rates have more than doubled since 1980.

BY 2014, 1.9 BILLION ADULTS WERE OVERWEIGHT, OF WHOM 600 MILLION WERE OBESE.

So, nutritious, delicious, satiating fats have been unfairly cast aside while unsatisfying, fat-inducing, health-ruining carbs have been allowed to run rampant. Moreover, the flavour that fat once imparted to our food has been replaced en masse by flavourants in general and in particular by an endless supply of sugar, carbohydrate in its most refined form. As a result, our grocery stores, refrigerators and kitchen cupboards are today filled with sweetened yoghurts, sugar-laden drinks, processed sugar-frosted cereals, flavoured crisps, crackers, breads, pastas and rice.

There is, however, good news. The Real Meal Revolution, with its low-carb high-fat real-food message, has by no means been a lone voice in the fight to overhaul global eating guidelines. New books, studies, articles and dietary guidelines appear by the week to endorse our position with sensible science, well-argued hypotheses and responsibly sourced evidence.

Even the US's Dietary Guidelines Advisory Committee – the descendant of the very committee that first adopted the diet-heart approach back in 1977 – has started to acknowledge the errors of its past. Its latest five-yearly guidelines, released in February 2015, have softened its stance on daily fat limits and completely dropped its long-standing recommendation to restrict consumption of dietary cholesterol. Most pertinently, fat is no longer its prime villain; that position is now, correctly in our opinion, taken by sugar.

On the next two pages you'll find a summary of the human journey: from health to obesity – and the turn back.

31

THE TIMELINE TO HUMAN OBESITY – AND RECOVERY

PRE-CIVILISATION

all communities are hunter/gatherers

1500 BC

civilisation in the fertile crescent boosted by farming of grains

Egyptians, "the eaters of bread", known to have suffered from "diseases of civilisation"

MID-17TH CENTURY:

sugar no longer considered a luxury, now a staple

1493

Columbus brings sugar cane to New World

C. 600

sugar spreads to Persia, production perfected

C. 500

sugar cane first processed into powder for easier use in food

1700

average Englishman consumes 1.8kg of sugar per year...

1800

... 8kg of sugar per year...

1862

William Banting, advised to avoid carbohydrates, goes on to popularise "Banting" diet

1900

... 45kg of sugar per year...

1870

... 21kg of sugar per year...

1860-1890

US Agricultural Revolution; boom in agriculture and farming

1953

Ancel Keys publishes paper claiming relationship between fat intake and rate of heart disease

1957

Drs Yerushalmy and Hilleboe review and refute Keys's study – review ultimately ignored

1966

1931 Nobel Prize winner for Medicine, Otto Warburg, claims "the prime cause of cancer is the replacement of the respiration of oxygen in normal body cells by a fermentation of sugar" – ultimately ignored

13 JANUARY 1961

Time magazine cover: Ancel Keys featured in a "Diet & Health" special

CONTINUED ON NEXT PAGE

1967
Harvard researchers paid by Sugar Research Foundation to overstate effects of saturated fats and cholesterol and refute real evidence against sugar

1972
Earl Butz appointed as US Secretary of Agriculture in hopes he will bring down food prices for Americans while increasing farmers' earnings

26 MARCH 1984
Time magazine cover: Two fried eggs with bacon strip arranged as sad face. Cover line: "Cholesterol. And now the bad news…"

1977
USDGA released advising Americans to consume 12 servings of grains and cereals per day. Global rates of obesity and diabetes increase "explosively" within five years

6 SEPTEMBER 1999
Time magazine cover: two fried eggs with melon piece arranged as smiley face. Cover line: "Cholesterol. The good news"

2000
Allessio Fasano discovers zonulin protein, revolutionising our understanding of gut health

2013
publication of bestselling *The Real Meal Revolution*: introduces LCHF eating en masse to South Africa

2007
publication of *Good Calories, Bad Calories* by Gary Taubes: critically analyses global nutritional guidelines, popularises concept of insulin resistance

2014
publication of *NYT* bestseller *The Big Fat Surprise*: makes the inarguable case for fat and against carbs, praised by *The Economist*, *The British Medical Journal* and other high-profile publications

2015
five-yearly USDGA update removes all limits on dietary cholesterol and reduces daily sugar recommendations

12 JUNE 2014
Time magazine cover: a curl of butter. Cover line: "Eat Butter. Scientists labelled fat the enemy. Why they were wrong"

NOT SO SWEET

Sugar's true culpability in the original myth-making that elevated carbohydrates and condemned fats was revealed in smoking-gun detail only very recently, with the revelation of internal sugar-industry documents detailing how, in 1967, three Harvard researchers were paid the equivalent of nearly $50,000 (£40,000) in today's value to falsify data. The documents from the Sugar Research Foundation, today known as the Sugar Association, were discovered by a researcher at the University of California, San Francisco and were published in *JAMA (Journal of the American Medical Association) Internal Medicine* in September 2016. They reveal that the researchers cherry-picked studies in a review of sugar, fat and heart research for the renowned *New England Journal of Medicine*, and "minimized the link between sugar and heart health and cast aspersions on the role of saturated fat". *The New York Times* reported at the time that "five decades of research into the role of nutrition and heart disease, including many
of today's dietary recommendations, may have been largely shaped by the sugar industry".

And they're still at it. It was reported in 2015 that Coca-Cola had spent millions funding research that seeks to play down the link between sugar and obesity, and in 2016 that a trade association representing several chocolate and confectionary brands in the US had funded a paper claiming that children who ate sweets weighed less than those who didn't. The moral of the story: always check the source of any nutrition and dietary finding.

WHERE ARE WE NOW?

Today the chronic health problems that emerged with the first human agriculture thousands of years ago have been exponentially exacerbated by widely available modern foods. The result is that many of us have been coerced by Big Food into the fat-storage state of energy metabolism, and permanently locked in by our hijacked appestats. What's more, we are still encouraged by many official dietary guidelines to continue fuelling ourselves in this exact way.

Though it's not quite as easy as flicking a switch (and different people can be more or less sensitive to carbohydrates), the success of the RMR diet lies in making the change from the fat-storage to fat-burning state, a process that is governed by the food we eat.

> "Once a fad diet, the safety and efficacy of the low-carb diet have now been verified in more than 40 clinical trials on thousands of subjects."
> **– SARAH HALLBERG OF INDIANA UNIVERSITY HEALTH ARNETT HOSPITAL AND OSAMA HAMDY OF HARVARD MEDICAL SCHOOL, WRITING IN *THE NEW YORK TIMES*, SEPTEMBER 2016**

For more...

- On the history of nutritional science in the late 20th century and its effect on obesity rates, we highly recommend *The Big Fat Surprise* by Nina Teicholz; or read the comprehensive *Good Calories, Bad Calories* by Gary Taubes or *The Real Meal Revolution*.
- On the most recent US Dietary Guidelines, see "The Scientific Report of the 2015 Dietary Guidelines Advisory Committee", available at health.gov.

1.3.2 THE FOUR HORSEMEN OF THE CARB-POCALYPSE

> "We've seen that there are four mechanisms directly associated with almost every lifestyle disease. Kill the horsemen, kill the disease."
> **– REAL MEAL REVOLUTION TEAM**

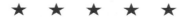

So, we know that we, as modern humans, are eating badly, which is making us overweight and unhealthy. But just how bad is it? What chronic diseases have been definitively linked to diet?

Before we get there, we need to take a look at the major mechanisms that are causing those links so we can understand them and make efforts to stop them. By now you'll be familiar with insulin resistance – the focus of *The Real Meal Revolution* – but there are three more mechanisms to consider that have received increasing coverage in nutrition and medical circles in recent years: gut problems, gluten sensitivity and chronic inflammation.

As with the various factors that make up the Pie of Life, to come (see p50), all four are often connected with or exacerbated by each other.

INSULIN RESISTANCE

"The single most important condition we need to treat is insulin resistance."

– Prof Tim Noakes

The first problem of living permanently in a carbohydrate-burning state is not hard to see: you put on weight. But a critical unseen problem is increased insulin resistance.

Each time you eat carbs, insulin is secreted to deal with the glucose. But the increasing amounts of insulin being secreted have less and less effect when it comes to burning the glucose in your system and preventing it from being stored as fat.

As with nicotine and other narcotics, the body gradually loses its sensitivity to insulin. Over time, ever more insulin is required to keep glucose levels under control when carbs are consumed. Meanwhile, the associated functions of high insulin levels continue, such as decreased metabolism (and thus increased lethargy) and increased appetite. The obesity cycle spins ever quicker and you suffer from ever more laziness and internal inflammation, which eventually becomes chronic inflammation.

Currently, traditional medicines "manage" related diseases but rarely, if ever, reverse them. "Take x for gout, y for depression and of course statins for high cholesterol…" Finally, when your blood results reveal you have developed type-2 diabetes, you will start having to assist your failing pancreas with medication and then externally injected insulin. Though this may seem like a solution, all it does is keep your blood glucose under control while the other effects of insulin, most notably the build-up of chronic inflammation throughout your body, simply get worse.

There are a couple of problems in conceptualising insulin resistance. First, you can't know how insulin resistant you are without getting tested – but we'll get to that. Second, it is something of an intangible notion because you never see insulin or its effects in action (except slowly, over time, so the association is forgotten). So if it helps, think of insulin resistance as "carbohydrate resistance". If you are "carb resistant" (insulin resistant), whenever you eat carbs – bread, pasta, chocolate, whatever – you are ingesting something your body can't process properly, and as a result you are more likely to suffer long-term ill effects.

For more on insulin resistance read...

■ *Good Calories, Bad Calories* by Gary Taubes or *The Real Meal Revolution*.

POOR GUT HEALTH

> "All disease begins in the gut."
> **– Hippocrates, c. 400 BC**

Hippocrates may not have been entirely right, but current medical thinking is increasingly emphasising the importance of the gut (intestines) and the links between digestion, mood and health. At RMR, we can verify that many, if not most, of our dieters who are overweight and insulin resistant appear to have poor gut health.

An enormous organ, the gut, often considered "the second brain", is a place of complex interaction between nerve signals, hormones and the gut flora. Upset it and the consequences can be numerous and nasty.

The small intestine is responsible for around 95 percent of the digestion and absorption of the food we eat. Nearly seven metres in length, it consists of internal folds that are in turn layered with miniscule protrusions designed to maximise the surface area available for absorption and digestion.

The total surface area exposed to both the nutritious and harmful things we consume has been calculated to be anywhere from the size of a badminton court to the size of a tennis court!

Key to the effective and healthy functioning of the small intestine is the symbiotic relationship it enjoys with our gut flora. These microorganisms line the intestinal wall by the trillions, forming a vital living interface between the partially digested food on the inside and the intestinal wall on the outside. Among other things, gut flora manufacture vitamins B and K, and act as an organ of the body by releasing hormones into the bloodstream.

As we have seen, hormones interact with the brain and signal the body to change its behaviour in response to a change in its environment. Irritable bowel syndrome (IBS) and its associated symptons such as constipation and bloating are now thought to directly affect our mood, contributing to major emotional shifts and even anxiety and depression (which in turn affect the gut).

Our gut flora also plays an important role in managing the body's metabolism, and it forms part of the body's immune system by making antigens from potentially harmful bacteria that the immune system can use to ward off disease.

Regardless of what diet you may sign up for, it is critical that it should take into account the healthy development and maintenance of your gut flora. Abrupt changes, such as a wildly fluctuating diet, the excessive use of antibiotics or the infestation of harmful bacteria, can seriously compromise this vital organ. Rebuilding and supporting the gut flora should be regarded as a foundational step to metabolic health and is therefore focused on in detail in Real Meal 2.0.

For more on gut health read...

■ *Gluten Freedom* by Alessio Fasano (Wiley, 2013) – or find his video lectures on YouTube.

GLUTEN SENSITIVITY

"Gluten is our generation's tobacco."
– David Perlmutter, *Grain Brain*

Lying adjacent to the layer of gut flora described above is your intestinal wall. This is lined with a selectively permeable membrane which, unlike a normal permeable membrane (like a coffee filter), is genetically coded to allow only a specific selection of chemicals, proteins, enzymes, fats and sugars through it into the bloodstream.

The cells that make up this membrane are bound together with organic bonds called "tight junctions" that usually require about 50 different biological processes to separate them, like a 50-step PIN code. The tight junctions would typically separate when the gut detects the trace of a new virus or toxin, allowing a microscopic trace of the toxin between the cells into the bloodstream before closing – the theory being that these trace elements teach the immune system how to fight the infections, similar to the way a vaccination works. This immune reaction causes minor inflammation but it is so short-lived you'd probably never know it happened.

The great gut disrupter is wheat (actually, gluten). Cultivated for only about 400 generations – and for many communities the exposure to it has been far more recent than that – wheat is seen by many doctors and dietary experts, whether LCHF proponents or not, as damaging to many, if not most, humans.

Wheat – along with barley, rye and other grains – contains gluten, of which gliadin is an important constituent. In the human gut, gliadin has the unique ability to activate a protein in the intestinal membrane called zonulin that miraculously unlocks the 50-step PIN code, separating the gut-lining cells and allowing random large molecules into the bloodstream: food particles, bacteria, stomach acids and pretty much any toxic (and non-toxic) substance that was destined to be flushed down the loo rather than absorbed into your body. This is known as leaky gut syndrome.

When all these foreign molecules make it into your bloodstream, your immune system responds as it would against those microscopic traces. The scene is thus set for a range of auto-immune diseases to potentially take hold in those genetically predisposed to them. Coeliac disease has long been identified as a hypersensitivity to gluten, but even those not predisposed to it may experience similar symptoms when consuming gluten-containing grains, the result of what's now known as non-coeliac gluten sensitivity. Leaky gut syndrome is now thought to be associated with type-1 diabetes, coeliac disease, Crohn's disease, irritable bowel syndrome and other digestion-related maladies, while gluten consumption is believed to negatively affect the brain, increasing the chances of Alzheimer's disease and other forms of senility.

For more on gluten sensitivity read...
- *Grain Brain* by David Perlmutter (Little, Brown and Company, 2013)
- *Gluten Freedom* by Alessio Fasano (Wiley, 2013)

CHRONIC INFLAMMATION

"Inflammation is the core behind virtually all modern disease."
– Gary Fettke, orthopaedic surgeon and anti-sugar campaigner

Inflammation in the body is designed to treat threats as they arise, not on a permanent basis. Although the inflammation in a specific area or organ might have been triggered to address one specific threat, when it becomes chronic, the side effects of inflammation can lead to a vast array of further conditions over time, with the body effectively turning on itself.

Although there are drugs to treat the illnesses associated with chronic inflammation, they cannot offer a cure because the core problem remains. As you age you must be prescribed more drugs in bigger doses, and in time you may need further drugs to treat the side effects of those drugs.

Today, chronic inflammation is recognised as a particularly dangerous threat to long-term health, and we believe it is a threat that needs to be dealt with at its root. It is a mechanism that we seek to address in Real Meal 2.0, both directly and by reducing the causes of it, such as insulin resistance and leaky gut syndrome.

WHAT IS CHRONIC INFLAMMATION?

Inflammation is one of your body's healing processes. If you sprain your ankle or stub your toe, your body responds by increasing blood flow to the area to provide more white blood cells and cellular "rebuilding materials"; as a result, it becomes swollen or inflamed. This process also disables movement in the area, offering protection and reminding you to look after it and let it heal.

Now imagine if you stubbed your toe, but instead of leaving it to heal in its inflamed state, you stubbed it every third day for the rest of your life: in time you would develop chronic inflammation – inflammation that persists for a long time or recurs regularly.

If you first stubbed your toe when you were 20 years old and kept on bashing it for the next 30 years, imagine the result of three decades of chronic inflammation on your fiftieth birthday: you may have had your toe amputated by then, or even your entire foot.

Think of inflammation throughout the rest of the body as similar.

For more on chronic inflammation...

■ Read *The Real Meal Revolution* and follow Professor Tim Noakes on Twitter: @ProfTimNoakes or find talks by Gary Fettke on YouTube.

SUMMARY

Insulin resistance, poor gut health, leaky gut syndrome and chronic inflammation are four interconnected mechanisms that fuel much – possibly the great majority – of our long-term maladies today.

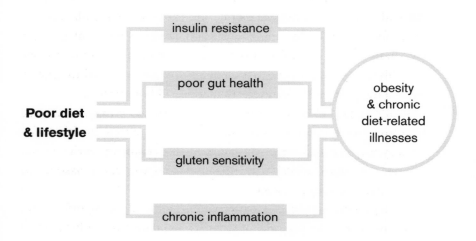

For a clearer illustration of what we're dealing with, including an overview of all the chronic illnesses that have been shown to be connected to diet, we need a new way of looking at it all: the volcano model.

1.3.3 FROM ICEBERGS TO VOLCANOES

In *The Real Meal Revolution*, Professor Tim Noakes described obesity, diabetes, hypertension and hypercholesterolaemia as merely the tip of the metabolic-syndrome iceberg. Out of sight were numerous conditions that hadn't been connected to dietary problems in the past but which have now been linked to insulin resistance (or "carbohydrate resistance", if you prefer).

Following Prof Noakes's lead, we have traced down the disease pathway from insulin resistance, as well as poor gut health, leaky gut syndrome and chronic inflammation, to come up with an even more complete overview of diseases and disorders associated with poor diet and lifestyle.

The process was time-consuming but relatively straightforward. We reviewed the work of renowned medical authorities – including specialists in the four mechanisms discussed above – and listed the conditions they have linked with excessive carbohydrate, sugar and gluten-rich grain consumption. We then cross-referenced their list of ailments with feedback we have received from our own customer base.

The result should, we feel, no longer be seen as an iceberg waiting to sink an unlucky ship. It is, rather, a volcano – powered by poor and self-perpetuating dietary and lifestyle choices – harbouring a red-hot core that can cause immense damage with an abrupt eruption once the lava has built up inside. And, like communities enjoying a peaceful life on the side of a sleeping volcano, it is rather too easy to ignore the wisps of smoke emerging from the top – until one day the top blows off.

When you write out the broad categories of diseases, disorders and conditions that have possible links with diet, the list looks like this:

Metabolic conditions

Cardiovascular disease

Neurological disorders

Muscular and skeletal diseases

Skin disorders

That may look concerning but perhaps doesn't have the sense of urgency we'd like to convey. For that, look right to see the many specific conditions within those categories… Suddenly it's all rather overwhelming!

The key to Real Meal 2.0 is to understand what's heating up the core of the volcano so we can take steps to cool it down and restore the health of the whole body.

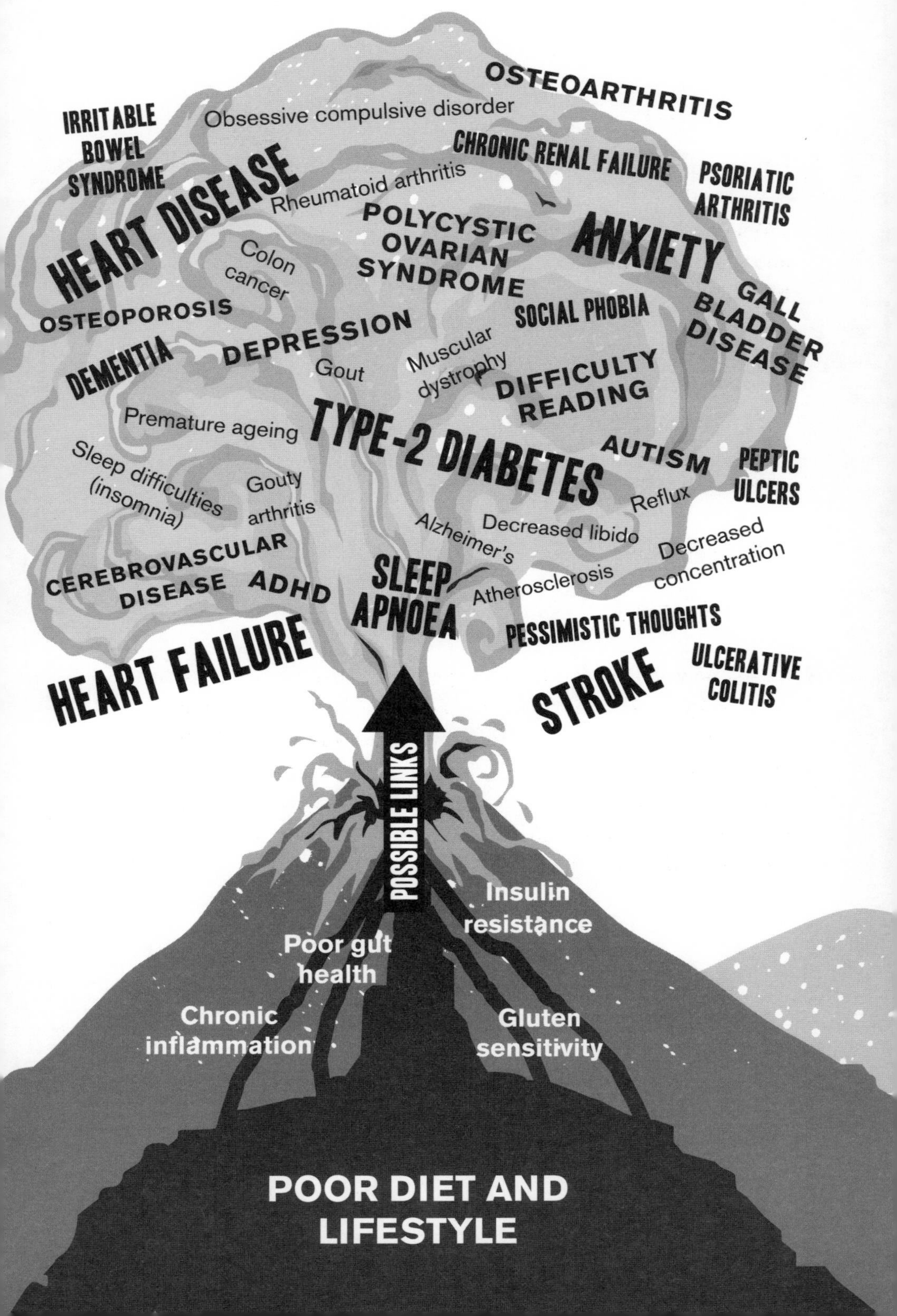

OSTEOARTHRITIS
IRRITABLE BOWEL SYNDROME
Obsessive compulsive disorder
CHRONIC RENAL FAILURE
PSORIATIC ARTHRITIS
HEART DISEASE
Rheumatoid arthritis
POLYCYSTIC OVARIAN SYNDROME
ANXIETY
Colon cancer
GALL BLADDER DISEASE
OSTEOPOROSIS
SOCIAL PHOBIA
DEPRESSION
DEMENTIA
Gout
Muscular dystrophy
DIFFICULTY READING
Premature ageing
TYPE-2 DIABETES
AUTISM
PEPTIC ULCERS
Sleep difficulties (insomnia)
Gouty arthritis
Reflux
Alzheimer's
Decreased libido
Decreased concentration
CEREBROVASCULAR DISEASE
ADHD
SLEEP APNOEA
Atherosclerosis
PESSIMISTIC THOUGHTS
HEART FAILURE
STROKE
ULCERATIVE COLITIS
POSSIBLE LINKS
Insulin resistance
Poor gut health
Chronic inflammation
Gluten sensitivity
POOR DIET AND LIFESTYLE

PART 2
REAL MEAL 2.0:
THE DIET
THE LIFESTYLE

2.1 THE PIE OF LIFE

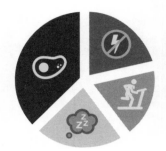

> "Our bodies are a physical representation of the way we have lived our lives. Each pound of flesh has its own story to tell of the choices we have made, the habits we have developed, our likes and dislikes, the relationships we have made with those we have met along the way.
> The only way to feel comfortable about your body and successfully keep off lost weight is first to become aware that being overweight and chronically unhealthy is a symptom of lifestyle imbalance. It is time to balance the system."
> **– LEAINE BREBNER, HEAD OF CONTENT, REAL MEAL REVOLUTION**

We've called this chapter "The Pie of Life", but to be clear: it's not about pie. Indeed, it's not even about food, except indirectly. But this chapter is critical because it offers an understanding of how your body works in its wider context so your decision to be more healthy and lose weight can become a sustainable reality.

Life is the key word here, and from it *lifestyle,* which, as we've identified already, is a fundamental pillar of Real Meal 2.0. Even though the Real Meal Revolution will always be built around following a real-food RMR diet, losing weight and being healthy isn't just about eating correctly; it's about recognising all the variables that affect the way your finely tuned body runs and getting them to work together in harmony.

WHY DO WE EAT?

No prizes for this: we eat because we're hungry. But why are we hungry? Natural hunger is the body's way of telling us to obtain energy to fuel our physiological functions. It's one of the basic drives we have from birth: we instinctively have to breathe, eat, sleep and be nurtured.

This is roughly how appetite/hunger *should* go:

A region of the brain called the appestat controls appetite. When blood-sugar levels fall below a certain point, messages are sent to the appestat; the appestat sends signals for the body to secrete certain hormones; and the hormones make us feel hungry. Once we've eaten enough, the process reverses and we feel full. Seems simple, but there is a complex balance of hormones that your appestat must manage to get this right.

As we grow older the appestat and the body's hormone levels can be affected by many other factors. The most notorious culprit, we believe, is the modern sugar- and carb-laden Western diet, which promotes insulin resistance. In so doing, it "hijacks" the appestat into not recognising when we've taken in enough fuel: we don't feel full so we eat more than we need and the excess food is stored as body fat. The understanding of this mechanism is at the core of the movement away from destructive high-carb foods.

There is, however, also a large psychological aspect to eating (and drinking), and we may come to eat for reasons besides hunger as a way to self-nurture; for example, as a coping tool to deal with sadness, stress or anger. Any situations that feel beyond our control are likely to stimulate stress hormones that can upset the delicate hormonal balance within the body and affect the appestat. Ever taken comfort in a large chocolate when you were feeling down, or "needed" a glass or two of wine at the end of a stressful day, or simply made yourself a sandwich because you were bored or procrastinating? Then it's happened to you.

Our bodies are designed for a simpler, more instinctive existence and in this complex modern world we encounter situations on a daily basis that can throw our system out of sync and encourage us to eat when, functionally, we don't need to.

FEEL RIGHT, EAT RIGHT

When our relationship with food is a healthy one, we don't obsess about it. We leave enough time between meals for our food to digest correctly and for all of our metabolic processes to receive the fuel they need to function correctly. We don't feel the need to snack and our bodies are happy.

In short, we feel right so we eat right.

When we don't feel right, we tend to eat badly. (Got Sunday blues? Order a pizza!) The powerful emotions associated with food are one possible explanation for this phenomenon. Memories of home, family, childhood, special occasions, safety, protection, abundance and giving are all often linked with food, and so food can become a nurturing crutch in times of need.

Comfort eating is a real phenomenon and it can be triggered by many things in today's fast-paced world.

HORMONES TO KNOW

There are eight main hormones (or types of hormone) that have an effect on body weight. The first four directly affect the appestat.

Insulin: the one we all know about; controls blood-sugar levels and promotes fat accumulation (among other things)

Ghrelin: the hunger hormone; increases appetite

Leptin: the satiety hormone; decreases appetite

Adiponectin: regulates fatty acid breakdown; promotes fat retention

The second four indirectly affect the appestat (among other things) by affecting the previous four hormones.

Cortisol: the "stress hormone"; released in response to stress, it raises blood-sugar and thus insulin levels

Adrenaline: the "fight or flight" hormone; usually released in response to danger, it prepares the body for imminent action by, among other things, raising blood-sugar and thus insulin levels

Thyroid hormones: regulate metabolism, among other things

Endorphins: uplifting hormones that depress pain and increase feelings of wellbeing

Too much work, too little sleep, rushing through meals, health problems, poor work-life balance, not making time to see friends and socialise, not making time for yourself and general stress are some of the major contributors to comfort eating. And here's the thing:

- They all affect your hormones in some way;
- You can do something about them.

PIECES OF THE PIE

The three critical pieces of the pie are exercise, sleep and stress management. Individually they are worthwhile pursuits, and thus we recommend each one in and of itself. If you can get more and better quality sleep, do it. If you can make time to exercise or de-stress, do it. But together they are exponentially more effective because they are interlinked and self-perpetuating. Sleeping well, exercising and de-stressing all make you feel better about yourself, raising self-esteem and self-worth. And when you feel better you will sleep better, be more motivated to exercise and find more fulfilment in activities that help you de-stress – a complex virtuous cycle. So, in giving attention to one, realise that you are giving attention to them all – and by improving one piece of the pie, it will be easier to improve the others.

Consider a (simplified) example of a negative lifestyle cycle. Mandy sees her doctor because she feels constantly exhausted and run down. He diagnoses her with elevated cortisol levels, which are affecting various aspects of her life.

Negative cycle, including high cortisol levels

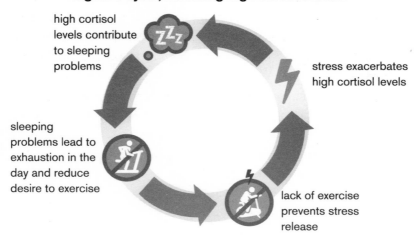

high cortisol levels contribute to sleeping problems

stress exacerbates high cortisol levels

sleeping problems lead to exhaustion in the day and reduce desire to exercise

lack of exercise prevents stress release

An effective intervention at any or all levels could change the cycle from negative to positive.

Turning a negative cycle into a positive cycle

balanced cortisol
levels lead to
better sleep

lower stress helps
balance cortisol
levels

better sleep
increases desire
to exercise

exercise helps
relieve stress

Besides affecting health, happines and quality of life in various ways, Mandy's original cortisol imbalance also affects her insulin levels and thus weight – and so we see how important the bigger picture is.

Now, let's look at each piece of the pie.

2.1.1 EXERCISE

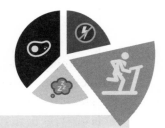

"Diet is Batman and exercise is Robin. Diet does
95 percent of the work and deserves all the attention;
so, logically it would be sensible to focus on diet."
– JASON FUNG, THE OBESITY CODE

... BUT...

"The higher your physical activity, the lower your insulin."
– Ted Naiman, physician

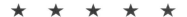

Exercise, like dieting, is one of those topics on which almost everyone has an opinion. And, like dieting, the best approaches are generally complex, specific to your individual needs and best ascertained from someone who knows what he or she is talking about (which unfortunately rules out many gym instructors...). We believe that exercise to assist with weight loss and health management is a topic that merits a book on its own; for now, the broad strokes must do.

The key to understanding exercise in the context of weight management is realising that it alone will make little difference to your weight. The idea that burning calories will allow you to shed pounds without any additional intervention has repeatedly been shown to be a myth. This has been proven in major studies and is evident in the increasing prevalence of obesity in countries that have a similarly increasing prevalence of exercise activity (often the result of well-intended but misguided government initiatives responding to the obesity crisis). Anecdotally, it is demonstrated in every story you've heard of someone starting an exercise programme and complaining a few weeks later that they hadn't lost any weight; it had just shifted. Possibly they'd even *put on* weight. (Happened to you?)

The studies do show, however, that *in conjunction with a dietary change* exercise certainly can help lose more weight than the dietary change alone. It makes you feel good about yourself and motivates you to take better care of yourself. What's more, exercise offers plenty of other health benefits and for those alone we highly recommend it.

THE HORMONAL EXPLANATION

Exercise can assist in weight loss by lowering levels of insulin and cortisol and increasing levels of endorphins. Insulin is the key to general weight loss, as per the LCHF hypothesis, so that's obviously a good start. Cortisol, the stress hormone, is similarly important in this instance, because it affects those insulin levels; by reducing your stress levels, you lower your cortisol levels and thus your insulin levels. And endorphins make you feel good about yourself, which improves your willpower and self-image and thus the likelihood that you'll stick to your diet.

But exercise can also *increase* your cortisol levels by stressing out your body over an extended period, which could in turn increase insulin levels. It also ups your appetite, which may be further affected by that extra stress, and suddenly the likelihood of a post-workout binge is on the cards...

So it's not a guaranteed weight-loss win unless you do it right.

WHAT TO DO

The greatest practical lesson we've learnt about exercise is this: don't dive into a new hectic routine right away. In fact, if you're not already exercising then don't start at the same time you start your RMR diet. There are various reasons why.

First, from a practical point of view, it's a good idea to keep track of diet and exercise variables separately so you can see their individual effects, which should help give you an idea of their importance to you. Second, when you start the RMR diet your energy levels may drop off a little, in which case you might struggle through a workout session, which can be demoralising. Third, your low energy levels may be exacerbated by intense exercise, in which case you may find yourself exhausted, sick or starving.

The fourth, and possibly most important, reason is the psychological element, usually linked to the points above. Making a major dietary change can be a tricky adjustment on its own; it just needs a bad week at work or a couple of days of flu to throw everything out of kilter and suddenly your new lifestyle doesn't seem manageable any more.

So: only start a new exercise regimen when you're 100 percent satisfied with your dietary changes, and even then keep it simple and sustainable, especially at the beginning.

If possible, train with a dedicated group of people who are at your fitness level, a strategy that gives more chance for success than exercising alone.

Some technical pointers:
- If weight loss is your goal, be sure to focus more effort on your diet than on your exercise.
- If possible, don't eat before you exercise.
- The more muscle you have, the more fat you can burn. In terms of specifics – what exercises to actually do – we like shorter, high-intensity workouts to build muscle mass, which increases your resting metabolic rate and improves insulin sensitivity without putting long-term stress on your body. If this interests you, follow Ted Naiman at BurnFatNotSugar.com or Ben Greenfield Fitness at BenGreenfieldFitness.com.
- That said, any exercise is usually better than none. Even though endurance work can place extended stress on your body, which can raise cortisol levels and may work against you (especially if you are a stressed person), there is great value in a long run, cycle or swim if it keeps you relaxed and sane. If it's beneficial to your emotional wellbeing, it's more likely to keep your programme on track. Just remember, you can't outrun a bad diet – and there are plenty of overweight marathon runners out there.
- After exercise your insulin levels will be low. Keep them there. Don't give yourself permission to down a sugary drink and eat a carb snack; rather drink water or bone broth and/or eat something high in fat or protein like a handful of nuts or a boiled egg.

EXERCISE SUMMARY

Exercise is an important part of managing your weight; it's just not as important as previously thought. Be honest and practical in your approach; start slowly and work out a realistic schedule. If you can look at exercise as a way to feel better and be healthy because of all the other important physiological benefits it provides, rather than as a short cut to dropping some excess pounds, you'll likely have more fun, get all those benefits *and* get the added weight loss.

For more, read...

■ "The Exercise Myth" in *The Obesity Code* by Jason Fung (Greystone, 2016); *The Art And Science Of Low Carbohydrate Performance* by Jeff Volek and Steve Phinney (Beyond Obesity, 2012); and *What the Fat? Sports Performance: Leaner, fitter, faster on low-carb healthy-fat* by Grant Schofield, Caryn Zinn and Craig Rodger (The Real Food Publishing Company, 2015)

2.1.2 SLEEP

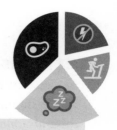

> "When a person sleeps less than seven hours
> a night there is a dose-response relationship between
> sleep loss and obesity: the shorter the sleep,
> the greater the obesity."
> – from "Extent and Health Consequences of Chronic Sleep Loss
> and Sleep Disorders" (see end of section)

★ ★ ★ ★ ★

Good-quality sleep is so important to us in so many ways, yet sleep deprivation may be as much an epidemic as the obesity crisis. Various studies, for example, estimate that about 35–40 percent of people in the US do not get sufficient sleep – very similar figures to that country's obesity rates.

Our collective sleep deficit is largely driven, it seems, by the realities of an increasingly frenetic world, in which demands on our time are numerous and difficult to prioritise and sleep is often equated with laziness or weakness. Whether due to supposedly justifiable demands such as work and socialising, or habitual and even addictive demands such as watching television and surfing the net, sleep is often the activity that suffers. And yet it is absolutely vital for our health and wellbeing – and it affects our weight both directly and indirectly.

THE HORMONAL EXPLANATION

The direct effect is, as might be expected, because of insulin. Sleep deprivation inhibits the body's ability to use insulin properly. "Metabolic grogginess" kicks in surprisingly quickly, with insulin sensitivity dropping by almost a third after just four days of disrupted sleep, according to a University of Chicago study. (Due to these potentially dramatic effects, sleep is considered by some to be as important as diet for people diagnosed with diabetes.)

Sleep also affects your body's levels of leptin and ghrelin, the satiety and hunger hormones: lack of sleep depresses the amount of leptin in your system and stimulates ghrelin, which makes you hungry. What's more, the after-hours message that you're feeling peckish is then more likely to be compounded by a bad eating decision because, by this stage, your cortisol levels will have been elevated for an extended period, which leads to an emotional need for rewards combining with poor self-control. Hence late-night snacking. And then day-time snacking. (Both bad.)

And there is a further layer of woe to add to this self-perpetuating toxic mix. Possibly the gravest effect of sleep deprivation is its impact on cognitive ability and decision-making – so much so that sleep deprivation is often compared to drunkenness. And what do people snack on when they're drunk? Exactly.

Most importantly, by making bad decisions you jeopardise your entire lifestyle.

WHAT TO DO

One of the paradoxes of contemplating the critical importance of sleep is that if you're not getting enough sleep you may not be thinking clearly enough to realise just how important it is. Trust us when we say, *get enough sleep*. This translates to a minimum of seven hours a night for anyone over the age of 18.

The first thing to do is the simplest and yet probably the hardest: prioritise sleep. Keep track of your sleeping patterns, honestly and accurately, and if you're getting less than seven hours a night then recognise you have a problem that needs fixing.

The fix may require drastic measures, including sleep therapy if necessary, but the most important change is the mental realisation that something must be done. Work less or socialise less, if needs be – and realise that by sleeping more you will do both of those activities better.

(The corollary is that too much sleep is also a bad thing: if you're aged 18–65 you're going for the Goldilocks zone of 7–9 hours.)

Some specific suggestions if you're struggling to get to sleep at night or aren't sleeping well:
- In general, sleeping pills are bad news; we recommend you avoid them. Certainly, do not self-prescribe. If you're really struggling, see a doctor.
- Naps are in. Only recently have the benefits of napping been properly studied, and it turns out they're numerous. If you can't get a good night's sleep, a 20- to 30-minute power nap the next day may be the next best thing. And even if you do sleep well at night, short naps may offer various benefits. Progressive corporates around the world are coming to recognise their importance, with the likes of Nike, Google and Apple providing napping facilities and encouraging employees to re-energise in the workplace. (If you do nap, ensure your naps don't affect your ability to get to sleep at night.)

- The numerous devices that dominate our lives these days, specifically our smartphones, have been identified as significant sleep disruptors. First, they encourage pre-sleep procrastination. ("I'm just going to watch one more episode / reply to one more email / spend five more minutes on Facebook.") And second, the blue-light wavelengths they emit, associated with daytime, are sleep suppressors. We recommend banning all screens from your bedroom beyond a certain time, or completely if you are not disciplined enough to follow a curfew. Either way, switch your device to Night Shift so that it automatically reduces the amount of blue light emitted after a certain hour. (The latest iPhones and iPads come with a Night Shift setting; otherwise use a free app such as Night Shift: Blue Light Filter.)
- Besides using modern electronics wisely, there are countless sleeping tips out there. Some of the better ones are: exercise, though not too late in the day (see previous section); reduce your stress levels (see next section); limit your alcohol and caffeine intake and don't drink coffee after lunch time; use guided meditation or prayer to clear your mind; wind down slowly in the evening, turning the lights down, listening to calming music, taking a bath and so on; follow a similar routine each night before bed so that both your body and brain recognise the signals that bedtime is approaching; ensure your bedroom is as quiet and dark as possible, and at the optimum temperature, which is lower than most people think, around 15–19°C.

SLEEP SUMMARY

Good sleep is non-negotiable if a) you want to be generally awesome, and b) you specifically want to keep the weight off. If you're well rested your metabolic rate will be higher than when you're tired, allowing you to burn more fat in your daily activities; the hormones that regulate your hunger will be more stable, along with your emotional state, making you less susceptible to unnecessary comfort eating; and your mental acuity and decision-making will be significantly sharper, allowing you to make better eating decisions and stick to your plans with more conviction.

For more...

■ Read *The Sleep Revolution: Transforming your life, one night at a time* by Arianna Huffington (WH Allen, 2016) for a comprehensive overview of the importance of sleep and how best to get it. We like the title; we believe the Real Meal and Sleep revolutions go hand in hand.

■ There are plenty of sleeping tips online; just be wary of the crackpot ideas. For some compelling science, including the effect of chronic sleep deprivation on weight and general health levels, see "Extent and Health Consequences of Chronic Sleep Loss and Sleep Disorders" from *Sleep Disorders and Sleep Deprivation: An unmet public health problem*, edited by Harvey R Colten and Bruce M Altevogt (National Academies Press, 2006), available at www.ncbi.nlm.nih.gov.

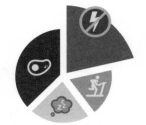

2.1.3 DE-STRESSING

> "If you're looking to lose weight, you should review possible ways to decrease or better handle excessive stress in your life."
> – Andreas Eenfeldt, low-carb specialist

We all know how bad stress is for us: it really is the bane of modern existence.

Stress has been blamed for just about every malady under the sun, from skin irritations and backache to viral infections and cancer; from high blood pressure and heart attacks to mental-health problems and premature ageing. And yes, weight gain is another. (As are digestive problems.)

Whether you're looking to lose a few pounds or not, dealing with stress should be an ongoing priority for your overall happiness. Of course, exercising (non-stressfully) and sleeping well contribute hugely to this – but you know that by now, right?

THE HORMONAL EXPLANATION

When we are put in stressful situations our bodies pump out high levels of cortisol and adrenaline, as well as endorphins to some extent. In our hunter-gatherer days this was the concoction needed when confronted by imminent danger. The blood supply to the muscles would increase, the heart's output would get a boost and our blood-sugar levels would spike so that we had a ready supply of fuel to burn. Then some kind of physical reckoning would take place: we'd either battle the bear (fight) or we'd run away as fast as our little legs could carry us (flight).

Today our bodies respond to all sorts of modern stimuli – be it driving in traffic, working on deadline, or shouting at your neighbour – with the instinctive stress responses of old, but they are seldom validated by a physical conclusion. As a result, all that pumped-up cortisol and adrenaline stays in our system longer than it should. Many of us are thus chronically stressed, with high cortisol levels keeping our insulin levels elevated and increasing the likelihood of us developing insulin resistance, among other things.

Over time both cortisol and adrenaline (indirectly) increase deposits of belly fat. This body fat in turn secretes leptin, which is supposed to prevent you from eating, but the higher the belly fat, the worse leptin works. In such cases it can actually end up working like ghrelin, the hunger hormone; this is known as leptin resistance – or you can consider it chronic hunger.

Needless to say, the more weight you put on the more likely you are to be chronically stressed, which means you're more likely to put on more weight because you're chronically hungry...

And as the sugar-sweetened cherry on top, stress can diminish thyroid function, which decreases basal metabolism and makes it even harder to lose weight.

F*%!ing stress!

RESTORING BALANCE AND RETURNING TO HAPPINESS

In certain ways, stress and stress management are a microcosm – or snapshot – of the greater lifestyle pie. There are many interconnected variables and there is an argument for including elements mentioned below, such as meditation, mindfulness and social interaction, as their own separate pieces of the pie. Certainly, there have been many books about and studies performed on these individual topics.

We have chosen to include them under the umbrella of de-stressing both for sake of ease and because they are different answers to the same question: how can we relax and be happy?

As with the lifestyle pie, we believe the answer lies in restoring balance to our lives – and to do this we need to address all of our Maslovian-like needs:

The need for survival: to eat, sleep and to feel safe;

The need for nurture, love and attention;

The need for belonging and connection;

The need to feel a sense of purpose, goals and meaning;

The need for independence and a sense of control;

The need for fun, stimulation and variety.

Here are a few suggestions:

- Address your eating habits, sleep problems and safety concerns (the first two should go without saying at this point...).
- Spend time on your close relationships, whether with your partner, family or friends.
- Make an effort to socialise and interact with people.
- Make time for yourself.
- Join a group, find a hobby and/or do something creative.

- Improve your skills.
- Use prayer, meditation, mindfulness, yoga, outings in nature or similar calming activities to gain control and confidence.

In short, do what makes you happy – in a constructive, positive way.

The exercises in the following section will help identify where to focus your time and energy.

DE-STRESSING SUMMARY

De-stressing will improve almost every health aspect of your life. Importantly, in the context of this book, it will also help you to lose weight. So take some time to self-assess and work out how best to manage your stress. You may have to make some hard decisions to better allocate your time and emotional energy, but it will be absolutely worthwhile.

For more...

- See www.chopra.com, read *A Practicing Mind* by Thomas M Sterner (New World Library, 2012) or *A Mindfulness Guide For The Frazzled* by Ruby Wax (Penguin, 2016), or ask your friends to recommend any book on de-stressing, mindfulness or meditation.

2.1.4 MEASURING YOUR PIE

> "Statistically, results from RMR dieters who track their progress are significantly better than results from those who don't."
> – MATT MURDOCH, HEAD OF ANALYTICS, REAL MEAL REVOLUTION

In this section we've considered the many variables that affect your weight and general health, though we've hardly touched on diet. For most people diet tends to be the largest piece of the pie, often significantly larger than the others combined, but this varies greatly from person to person. The amount of attention you should consider giving each piece depends entirely on you.

The chart on the opposite page, adapted from a number of sources and references, offers a visual representation of the potential for various lifestyle interventions to change your insulin levels, thus affecting your weight and health. Note that this is a conceptual illustration; the y-axis measurements of insulin and fat burning/storage are not to scale.

OVERHAULING YOUR INSULIN LEVELS

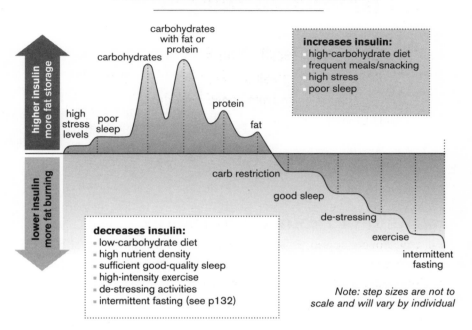

LIFESTYLE PIE CHARTS

As creatures of variety, we need different things in our lives to be fulfilled and happy. This applies to eating different foods, keeping our minds active with different hobbies and projects, and keeping our days varied. The lifestyle pie tables on p169 are designed to open your mind to the way you spend your time.

To work out what aspects of your life you may want to focus on, we advise keeping track of your activities over the course of a week, and if necessary over several weeks. In particular, we recommend doing this as part of Observation week, the first step of the phased approach (see p75 and on). You can fill it in every day or record what you got up to at the end of the week. For more digital tools, see RealMealRevolution.com.

The consistently interesting feedback we get on this exercise is that the statistics often don't correlate with a person's image of themselves. Many people think they are more active than they are. Or they don't realise how much time they spend watching TV compared to socialising, for example. When the lifestyle pie chart is created, people often realise they are not living the life they want to be living.

MEASURING YOUR PIE SUMMARY

The way you spend your time and who you spend it with is undeniably linked to your health, weight and wellbeing. Later in the book, when you set your goals, the results of this exercise should play an important role in working out what those goals are. Consider the time you spend doing activities and set goals to do more of the things you like and less of the things you don't like. Similarly, look to spend more time with the people you want to spend time with. Perhaps you could even set group goals with some of them.

Whatever you learn from this exercise, the intention is to help you bring balance to your Pie of Life. Make sure you're getting enough exercise and sleep. Manage your stress levels by managing your time effectively and looking after yourself. You will likely find that these small changes work together in the complex system of your life to set you on the path to weight loss and good health.

See the Awesome checklist on p142 to troubleshoot your exercise, sleep and stress if you're struggling with any of them.

General chapter resources:

- *50 Ways To Soothe Yourself With Food* by Susan Albers (New Harbinger Publications, 2009)
- *The Obesity Code* by Jason Fung (Greystone, 2016)
- *What Are You Hungry For?* by Deepak Chopra (Ebury Publishing, 2015)

2.2 EATING RIGHT

Reduced to its simplest and most fundamental level, the RMR diet is about switching the body's energy metabolism from a preference for carb-burning to a preference for fat-burning. Real Meal 2.0 adds several layers of complexity to this core idea, both externally in incorporating the various pieces of the Pie of Life, and within the fourth piece itself, the Diet, by adding a phased approach to LCHF eating and offering a clearly delineated list of foods to be embraced, avoided and wary of.

So:

The Science – check.

The Lifestyle – check.

Now it's time to get into the meat of things, the Diet.

Time to get awesome.

2.2.1 INTRODUCING THE PHASED APPROACH

The problem with fad diets is they don't work in the long run. You cannot simply change what you eat for a short period of time, reach a goal weight (if you do, in fact, reach it) and expect to maintain that weight forever. This has been repeatedly proven in clinical studies, and we've seen plenty of anecdotal evidence in our work.

This is one reason why we've spent time on the Pie of Life and emphasise Real Meal 2.0 as a lifestyle, not just a diet. It's also why we've introduced a new phased approach to our diet, a structured way to manage the transition from your previous dietary and health behaviours to a way of eating that offers amazing and sustainable results and forms the basis of a new, life-changing lifestyle.

THE RMR LEARNING CURVE

In the first *Real Meal Revolution*, we offered basic dietary information (along with important science and delicious LCHF recipes), but we left some readers punching in the dark when it came to the practicalities. This chapter introduces the steps we have arrived at after analysing our members' success, expert advice and the latest research into weight loss, anti-inflammatory dietary interventions, behavioural change management, adult education, habit formation and personal transformation. All the basics are in these pages, and the RealMealRevolution.com website provides a comprehensive set of tools to help calculate your goals and keep track of your progress.

There are four phases in the Real Meal 2.0 diet: Observation, Restoration, Transformation and Preservation. Each has a specific purpose. The first two are designed to get your mind and your digestive system fighting fit and ease you into weight loss; this will enable you to limit potential side effects, clear your mind and prepare your body for sustainable weight loss over the long term. The third focuses on strict low-carb eating for maximum fat burning; this is where the most dramatic action happens, though it is not necessarily the most critical phase. And the all-important fourth phase allows you to maintain the great foundation you've now built – for life.

Observation will give you a clear understanding of your current dietary and health state of affairs, helping to identify the elements of your lifestyle that could be contributing to your weight and poor health. Though it will require some active work, you won't be making any dietary changes at this point.

Restoration is effectively a light introduction to the RMR diet. This is where you get your head around a life without gluten, sugar and refined carbs – similar to the eating guidelines in *Raising Superheroes*. A focus on repairing your gut lining by including fermented and nutrient-dense foods contributes to the main aim of this phase: to prepare your body and mind for the next phase while avoiding potential side effects.

Transformation is the liberating phase where you will likely lose the most weight and see the most dramatic improvement to your health. This phase sees you reducing your carbs down to ketogenic levels.

Note: Some RMR dieters lose weight steadily enough during Restoration that they don't ever need to enter Transformation; they can skip straight to Preservation.

Preservation is not so much a phase as the rest of your life. Once the first three phases of Real Meal 2.0 have made a significant impact on your health, your weight and your life, all that is now required is for you to maintain your good eating habits. By the time you reach this phase you will have a clear understanding of your carbohydrate tolerance (insulin resistance) and your repaired gut biome will simply need regular fertilising and watering.

Note: Some people may never reach the Preservation phase due to severe insulin resistance or other health problems; as a result, Transformation is effectively their preservation phase. In contrast, for people who don't need to lose weight in the first place, we recommend Preservation from the get-go for sustained weight maintenance and optimum health.

A NOTE ON CHANGING BEHAVIOUR

Of the various adult learning methodologies available today, we agree with those experts who have found that the Jennings & Fuse 70:20:10 learning methodology, based on that latest research in adult education, gives the most effective, long-lasting results.

The justification for the Jennings & Fuse model is research that revealed that almost no education programmes (1 in 20) include pre-learning and very few (1 in 10) include follow-up learning. Analysis of the adult learning programmes that work the best showed that the most successful format was broken down into approximately 10 percent pre-learning (preparation and reading prior to the courses starting) and 20 percent actual learning (time spent on the course), with a full 70 percent dedicated to follow-up or ongoing monitoring and assessment.

(Coincidently, this habit-forming or adult-learning ratio is identical to the ideal macronutrient ratio we aspire to during Transformation.)

Having dealt with thousands of RMR dieters, these stats make perfect sense to us, with Observation equating to pre-learning, Restoration and Transformation to actual learning/doing, and Preservation to ongoing monitoring and assessment.

The moral of the story:
TO WORK IN THE LONG RUN
YOUR DIET MUST BECOME A LIFESTYLE.

2.2.2 THE LISTS: WHAT TO EAT

The original *Real Meal Revolution* introduced the concept of The Lists, an easy colour-coded way to get to grips with the foods to be embraced (Green), wary of (Orange) and Avoid (Red) when following the RMR diet.

In the intervening years we've continuously revised and fine-tuned the lists by following the latest science, taking on board extensive member feedback and considering the negative and positive health effects of foods that go beyond mere carb count. So there may be Green-listed foods with higher carb (and even sugar) content than those on the Orange or Red lists, but be assured that there is sound dietary and nutritional reasoning for this.

We've seen what works at various phases of the diet and added several shades of usability to it – so now we have a Green, Orange A and Orange B, Light-Red, Red and even Grey list.

Foods on the Light-Red list are high in carbs but contain no gluten or sugar and are not considered unhealthy in all other respects. For most RMR dieters who reach Preservation and wish to up their carb intake, Light-Red foods can be eaten without health concerns, though they must be monitored to see whether they affect weight.

Foods on the Grey list are those we have mixed feelings about. They may not be high in carbs or sugar, but they may not be real and they may not be healthy, so we have left them without endorsement for the time being.

More about all the colours, new and old, ahead.

GREEN
WHENEVER

Eat all Green foods until satisfied during all phases.

"Until satisfied" can be a difficult term to gauge, especially initially. If your appestat is out of sync, you may overeat out of habit; this will come right in time.

In short, the Green list includes:
- All naturally fermented foods (e.g. sauerkraut and pickles) – we recommend a portion of these foods to be included on a daily basis (see p207 onwards);
- Selected vegetables;
- All seafood, meats, poultry, game, eggs and offal;
- All naturally cured meats like pancetta, Parma ham, coppa, bacon, salami, biltong, jerky;
- All animal-derived fats and nut and fruit oils;
- All caffeine-free, sugar-free and additive-free drinks, homemade naturally flavoured waters (and, of course, water);
- All vinegars, flavourings and condiments, provided they are Real Meal friendly or homemade (and thus free from sugar, preservatives and vegetable oil);
- All hard cheeses such as mature cheddar, pecorino, parmigiano.

ORANGE (A AND B)
IN LIMITED QUANTITIES, DEPENDING ON WHICH PHASE YOU'RE IN

Orange foods generally contain more carbs but are otherwise healthy. We've refined this list to exclude certain foods during Transformation. The addition of dairy to the list is a sometimes controversial one, as dairy can prove problematic for certain people – see p149.

ORANGE A

Eat until satisfied during Observation and Restoration and cautiously during Preservation. During Transformation follow the limitations for food types and eat only one item per day.

In short, the Orange A list includes:
- All fresh dairy products, such as milk, cream, yoghurt, cream cheese, mozzarella and other soft cheeses;
- Non-dairy milks like almond, rice and coconut milk;
- Starchy vegetables – limited to half an upside down handful per day during Transformation (about a quarter cup, depending on the size of your hands).

ORANGE B

Eat until satisfied during Observation and Restoration and

cautiously during Preservation. Prohibited during Transformation.
- All dried legumes – best prepared soaked before cooking or sprouted;
- Coffee and caffeinated tea;
- All fruits.

LIGHT-RED
HARDLY EVER, MAYBE NEVER

Eat freely during Observation. Prohibited during Restoration and Transformation. Eat sparingly, or as often as your body will allow, during Preservation. (Think of it as "you wouldn't say no at a dinner party".)

Recognising our differing levels of insulin resistance, the Light-Red list makes some foods that were previously on the Red list available to certain people at certain times, including various (gluten-free) grains. It also includes some high-carb foods, like honey and pure maple syrup.

In short, the Light-Red list includes:
- Homemade vegetable juices and smoothies, dried fruits, honey and maple syrup;
- Gluten-free grains and gluten-free grain products;
- Gluten-free flours.

RED
NEVER EVER

*Eat freely during Observation. Then do your absolute best
to never eat them ever again.*

Red is the NO-YOU-CAN'T-EAT-THIS list. These are the foods
that have driven the obesity epidemic of recent decades,
including foods that are high in sugar and carbohydrates and/or
are unhealthy in some way. We strongly advise you to avoid all
the foods on this list.

In short, the Red list includes:
- All flours and all breads made from grains containing gluten;
- All cereals, biscuits, bars, crackers, chips and crisps;
- All juices, soft drinks, energy drinks and any drinks containing
  sugar;
- All seed oils and shortenings (virgin or not);
- All highly processed meats, polonies etc;
- All sweets that aren't RMR diet-friendly;
- All confectionery and (non-dark) chocolates (including
  "protein", "energy", "breakfast" or "snack" bars);
- All artificial sweeteners, sugar replacements, malts, blossoms,
  nectars and fructose;
- All food that contains added sugar;
- All deep-fried foods.

GREY
IT'S A GREY AREA...

Your call.

The Grey list is made up of foods, drinks and additives that we're neither confident in giving blanket permission nor blanket denial. Each item may have a place in your life or culture but we don't believe they are strictly beneficial for your health. They may, however, be beneficial for your sanity, which can be equally important – we will leave that decision to you. Alcohol is the obvious one here – see p152. See also p190 for more on supplements.

Please be aware that regardless of your interest in the consumption of these items, the carb count is something you will have to keep your eye on.

In short, the Grey list includes:
- Soy and tofu;
- Sugar-free or low-carb treats;
- Natural sweeteners such as erythritol, stevia and xylitol;
- Alcohol;
- Protein shakes and most supplements.

For more... See the full lists in colour (as a pull-out section) and black and white (from p236) at the back of the book for easy access. Also see realmealrevolution.com/real-food-lists.

A NOTE ON FATS

Now that we've introduced the List, let's clarify our position on fat. The RMR diet is low-carb high-fat, so fat is good, right?

In short, yes.

As we say in the first line of the book: fat is the best energy source for humans. Though it has been condemned for decades, good fats are perfectly healthy, and certainly far preferable to carbohydrates.

But, as with most things in life, too much of a good thing can be a bad thing, and perhaps the original *Real Meal Revolution* was not clear enough on the matter. To clarify then: the main reason the RMR diet is described as high-fat is because it is *not* a low-fat diet. Eating slices of butter in a butter sandwich sprinkled with butter (while drinking bulletproof coffee) is NOT a good idea. Following an LCHF lifestyle is not an excuse to go pouring extra fat on all your food.

The nuance lies in the difference between Restoration and Transformation. The goal is to get the body into a fat-burning state, then let it burn the fat that is already in the body. To achieve this in Restoration, and especially for people accustomed to a very low-fat diet – i.e. they've been taking in their calories almost exclusively in the form of carbohydrates – it may be necessary to make an effort to eat extra fat to get used to eating and burning fat.

In Transformation, the phase in which you're likely to lose the most weight, you'll want to make sure you are burning your own fat. This means dropping your fat intake to a point where you're satiated but not consuming more than you can burn off.

As LCHF guru Steven Phinney explains it:

"When you go on a weight-loss, ketogenic diet, you *can* eat less fat on your plate because you're burning the fat that comes from your inside. It comes from your love handles and hips and so on. When burning your own body fat, it looks like it's a high-protein diet. But the scales go down because the body's burning its own fat stores."

In fact, you only need to significantly up your fat consumption when you reach a body fat percentage of 20 percent or less. Some RMR dieters may never need to increase fat intake significantly while maintaining excellent blood and weight-loss results.

Bearing in mind that they can vary significantly from individual to individual, these are our broad fat-intake guidelines for the Real Meal 2.0 phased approach:

Observation – as much as you feel the need to.
Restoration – up to two thumbs of liquid or solid fat per meal.
Transformation – according to online ratios or no more than one thumb of liquid or solid fat per meal.
Preservation – as needed.

For your customised guidelines use the fat-intake calculator at RealMealRevolution.com. That said, for many RMR dieters life is too short to count and weigh every meal. Unless you're a perfectionist, roughly follow the guidelines above and, as always, be aware of how your body reacts.

2.3 THE MENTAL APPROACH

2.3.1 GOAL SETTING

> "An archer cannot hit the bull's-eye
> if he doesn't know where the target is."
> – ANONYMOUS.

The greatest diet in the world – no matter how much research you've done; no matter whether it incorporates a holistic lifestyle approach or not – will end in failure if it's not properly implemented. This is the practical side of human behaviour that transcends the science – and it's something we've learnt over and over at Real Meal Revolution, both in our own personal stories and in the many stories of those who have worked with us.

The first thing you have to do is set a goal – not that hard. Then you have to lock yourself into that goal and give yourself no option other than succeeding – and that *is* hard.

We cannot emphasise enough how important effective goal setting is.

If you're comfortable with your own goal-setting techniques that's a good start, and perhaps you'd like to skip straight ahead to section 2.4. If not, we recommend RMR's battle-proven two-part goal-setting process, which uses a very specifically structured set of goals and a locking-in method we call The Summons that's designed to create accountability and motivation.

YOUR GOAL

Goal setting is easy if you follow some basic rules. If you don't, it's rather a big waste of time.

Goals that are likely to remain unachieved might be "I want to eat healthily and lose weight" or "I'd like to feel comfortable in a bikini this summer". These are worthy aspirations but poorly articulated goals.

At RMR we suggest adopting the SMART goals model. SMART means:

SPECIFIC   Is it clearly explained?
MEASURABLE   Can it be measured, and what is the measurement?
ACHIEVABLE   Is it actually achievable and realistic?
RELEVANT   Is it relevant to what you want out of life?
TIME-BOUND   Is there a specific date and time that this goal will be achieved by?

Specific, *Achievable* and *Relevant* are generally straightforward when it comes to dieting, but give them due thought. Are you aiming to lose weight or get healthier or get fitter or look more attractive – or all of the above? Are you being realistic and sensible? (Remember, sustainable health and weight loss don't happen overnight.) Are your goals relevant to you and the life you lead? (We believe that most weight- and health-related goals are, but consider the specifics.)

Measurable and *Time-bound* are absolutely critical. Setting a SMART goal requires clear-headed forward thinking. There must be a tangible number or result that you can visualise, day in and day out, as you head towards it. Nothing must be left to the imagination. Ask yourself:

What measurement will make you happy?

Is it a certain number of inches off the waist?

Is it a particular blood reading – your blood-insulin levels, for instance – that will signify better health?

Is it a specific time for a race or running/cycling/swimming distance?

Is it a bench-press weight or the number of pull-ups you can do in a minute?

Is it the disappearance of back pain when playing golf or bloating after meals or foggy head in the morning?

Is it the number of times you poo in a day?

What is your deadline?

On which day does summer start for you? Pick a date and time.

Once you have those answers, define your goal in the form of an "I" sentence – a sentence about you – that is written in the first person, as though it has already happened.

"It is 1 December 2017 and I have a 34-inch waist."

Now, you have a date in the calendar and a number you can continuously repeat to yourself or visualise while you are going about your day. Notice that there is also no emotion attached to it. In time it will simply become a destination.

Now, serve yourself The Summons.

THE SUMMONS

"You can't be ready to commit. You must commit to be ready."
– JONNO PROUDFOOT

Although I understand that different people may want to go about setting and focusing on their goals in different ways, I feel so strongly about this next step (here and in any significant goal-setting process) that I've returned in the first person to try to convey the importance of it.

The way you feel about yourself is the single most important thing in your life for happiness and self-fulfilment, and you are now setting a goal for that. Even if you don't use this specific technique in the end, do please realise just how critical the psychological element of accepting a change of lifestyle is. If you want to do it right – and reap the rewards – you need to commit mentally and emotionally to the process.

Breaking up

We've said it all along: overhauling your health and weight is about lifestlye, not just diet, so when you do it there are going to be secondary effects beyond your kitchen. It's complicated, a lot like breaking up with a partner. It's not just about the two of you (you and your food); it's about who you used to hang out with (eat and drink with). No-one who isn't absolutely involved in your life is going to sympathise much. Your friends' lives are going to carry on as before. They'll eat what they want and you may hate them for it. When you complain about your new stupid diet they'll ask why you broke up in the first place, and when the dessert order comes you'll feel like you're watching all your friends hook up with your ex...

I'm painting a depressing picture here to illustrate just how tough a change of lifestyle can be, and what it takes upfront to give yourself the best chance of success.

The first thing to realise is it's very unlikely to work in isolation, so you're going to have to make some (non-dietary) changes in your life. You're going to have to involve the people who matter to you in your goal, and if necessary you may need to see less of certain people who don't share your approach to food and eating – or see them in different ways. A friend you usually have tea and cake with might become the new friend you go on walks with, for instance.

To do this effectively, we call on The Summons, which uses different tiers of accountability to assist you in the process. Let me explain.

A summons is a document issued by the courts; it details the particulars of a claim someone has made against you. Once you've been served with a summons you immediately have two tough options to choose between: you can spend time and money to defend yourself in court or you can do nothing, in which case, the court enforces the charge and puts the might of the law on your tail. You have no other option; you are stuck between a rock and a hard place. Whatever path you take it's going to be a difficult one. (Of course, we recommend defending yourself!)

Similarly, in committing to your diet you need to issue your own summons to give yourself two difficult tough options, rather than having one difficult one (stick to your new eating plan) and an easy opt out (quit). The first tough option is established:

following a new diet and lifestyle. Now you must make the second as important: locking yourself into the diet with a commitment that is more painful to endure should you fail than the diet itself.

When Thane and I swam the Mozambican channel, we were lucky enough to inadvertently issue our own summons. By the time we hit the water, we had two corporate sponsors who had invested money in us; we had a swimming coach and swim school that had spent time and offered facilities to train us for free; we had approximately a hundred friends and family between us who had been told in great detail over a rather lengthy period what we were attempting to do; we had a committed crew on the boat who were taking a month out of their lives for the sole purpose of supporting us; and we had thousands of children who would benefit from the money we hoped to raise. The weight of expectation on our shoulders turned out to be more daunting than the months of training and weeks of actually swimming 285 miles (459km) to Madagascar.

There were so many just-throw-in-the-towel moments on that trip that we lost count, but we were so desperately locked into our goal that dying seemed preferable to failing and then having to face everyone. Letting down the people we had invited into our adventure would have been far more painful than any amount of swimming we had to do.

In issuing your own summons you need to place yourself in a similar situation: between the rock of trying to start a difficult new phase in your life (it gets easier!) and the hard place of letting down those you had committed to. (The good news for you is you don't have to worry about sharks and jellyfish.)

This step takes great courage for some. If you've ever had a goal or dream that you thought people might laugh at if you told them,

I feel for you. But there is a paradox in not telling them. Because one of the best ways to increase your chance of success is by including and engaging with others.

HERE ARE TWO SCENARIOS

It is exactly one year until a specific ultra-marathon. Two people, John and Mary, have decided to run it next year. Although they are of equal fitness and the idea of a marathon is terrifying for both of them, they each adopt a different approach.

On the day that entries open, though it is a year until race day, Mary goes online and buys an entry. She tells her friends and family she's doing it. She joins a running club and tells the coach what her goal is, and asks him if he can give her pointers. She spots runners in the group who have the same goal and asks them questions about how they're going about it; she also tells these runners what she's doing. She even approaches her friends and family to sponsor her run in aid of a local charity, and she encourages her running buddies to do the same.

On the flip side, John tells himself he's going to enter at a later date because there are always spots available. He'll hold out until the day before to buy his ticket. He doesn't tell any of his friends and family what his goal is because he's worried about being *that guy*. He thinks groups are lame and doesn't fancy himself as a joiner. He also isn't sure he wants to be seen as "a runner". He decides he's going to go it alone and train himself. He doesn't ask for help. He doesn't like to put anyone out of their way and he also feels a bit silly asking advice on a simple thing like running, so he also avoids any kind of coaching. It doesn't occur to him to run the race in aid of anything or anyone.

Imagine John and Mary six months later. It's the middle of winter. It's pouring with rain outside. John and Mary's friends are out having a great time drinking in the pub and playing board games, but they have this marathon to train for so they're trying to stay on the straight and narrow. They've each suffered a few injuries and they're missing their families as a result of all the time they're spending running.

As the winter endures, who do think would find it easier to cop out of the race?

The answer is simple: John.

John is not accountable to anyone to complete the race. He hasn't told anyone. He hasn't joined with anyone. He has asked no-one for help, so no-one has invested time and effort into helping him. He hasn't offered to help anyone in running the race. He hasn't paid for his entry yet, so there isn't even a financial fallout.

Conversely, Mary almost has no choice. She's already paid for her entry. She has asked her coach for extra help on the side, creating an expectation on his front for her to succeed. Remember, coaches succeed through their students' success: Mary's completion of the marathon means almost as much to her coach as it does to her. Mary has also told her friends and family that she's training. They'll give her a hard time about not spending time with them but they will respect her for putting in the work. Mary also has a group of peers she has been training with who are going through the same thing. So even though it's really tough to leave the party early, when she gets up early the next morning to make her running group she'll be among people going through the same thing as her. And she's now raised enough pledges for her worthy cause to further motivate her.

As a result of the steps Mary took at the start of her journey, she has locked herself into a much harder shell of accountability to break out of than John has. In fact, it would take a major injury or life event to knock Mary off track.

Mary's approach can be broken down as follows:

- She committed long before she was ready (by paying and entering the race).
- She told people.
- She joined a group.
- She asked someone for help.
- She made her goal about helping others.

If we take Mary's approach to creating accountability around our goals, we would have a far higher chance of success. Different challenges require different forms of accountability.

The people you tell

Occasionally those closest to you may not be as supportive as you would expect or like them to be. When you declare your ambition to do something that they feel might be bigger or better than them, you challenge the belief they have of themselves, and that may trigger a negative response. When you tell someone about your goal and they talk it down, laugh or try to discourage you, it's often because they are feeling threatened or insecure.

Quite often the people who are closest to you will make it easy for you to quit because you quitting will make them feel better about their own health choices. In addition, nobody likes to see their friend struggling. They will make excuses for you to drop out so they can be the friends who "helped you". Unfortunately, the accountability you have to your loved ones is often bittersweet and may only return dividends once the post-achievement dust has settled.

The people who you join

When you join any support group you become part of something that you benefit from, just as the people in the group will benefit from your participation. When you look to your left and your right and see people suffering next to you, you will naturally feel more motivated. Likewise, the people to the left and the right of you will look at you and feel the same sense of motivation knowing that you are suffering with them. When you feel great, it's easy for you to attend a group and it's likely that your group will benefit hugely from you being there. Equally, when you're feeling terrible, you will benefit hugely from being with other people in your group. You might not think it, but you are just as important to the group as the other people in it. Watching others succeed is a source of inspiration and motivation, and when others see you succeed you will be a source of inspiration to them.

The person you ask for help

When you ask someone for help, you are asking them to invest a precious commodity – their time or effort – into you as a person. Regardless of whether or not you are paying for the help, your positive results will give both you and that person satisfaction.

Asking someone who is trained to help people feeds that person's purpose. There is nothing more flattering than being asked for help, even if it is your business. There is also nothing more rewarding than giving help that yields results. When you ask someone for help, you might think you are making them accountable, but you are actually making yourself accountable to them to achieve what you set out to achieve. If you don't achieve your goal then the person who has helped you has effectively failed – and that's on you.

The people you commit to helping

When you make your goal about helping other people, you become accountable to the people you intend to help.

Being motivated by charity is the obvious way to help others when you set yourself a goal – whether it is a local pledge at the office or online, or a bigger event with corporate sponsors – but you needn't look that far afield. It may be a promise to climb a mountain with your family or simply go on a hike with your child on her birthday. Whatever you choose, the gesture of offering your help – your promise – to another puts an onus on you to come through for them. The web of accountability thickens.

In the end you are accountable to everyone: yourself, your friends and family, your training partners, your coach or adviser, and the people you've offered to help.

GOAL-SETTING SUMMARY

To achieve greatness – or Awesomeness – of any sort you need to start with a very specific goal. Visualise the goal and lock yourself into achieving it to such an extent that the possibility of failure is more painful than the process itself. If you commit without being ready, tell people, join people, ask people for help and commit to helping people, your odds of success are drastically improved.

Here are the five elements to goal-setting and achievement, using The Summons technique:

- Commit by writing your SMART goal in an "I" sentence.
- Tell people.
- Join people.
- Ask people for help.
- Help people.

While you go through the remaining sections, give some thought to who you want to tell, who you might want to join on this crusade, who you might ask for help and how you could possibly make this about helping or benefiting someone else.

2.3.2 GETTING TO AWESOME!

> "There has got to be more to life than just being really, really, really, ridiculously good-looking."
> – DEREK ZOOLANDER

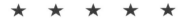

For many dieters, weight loss can become an obsession. But there is a major problem evident in the name itself: *weight* loss. Often an anxious daily fret on the scale to see how many pounds may have disappeared or reappeared, weight loss as an end in itself can be a dangerous goal.

We prefer to keep the focus on becoming healthier and feeling better – what we call Getting To Awesome. Part of this process, of course, involves losing weight, but more importantly, you want to lose fat, lose inches in the right places, improve your lifestyle and feel better about yourself. When you look in the mirror and you're happy, then you're probably at Awesome.

WORKING OUT YOUR IDEAL WEIGHT AND HIP-WAIST RATIO

Monitoring weight loss is most important when you start the RMR diet, particularly if you're very overweight or obese. Seeing the pounds and inches falling off week by week is an indicator that you're on the right track and a huge motivator to keep going.

The practical trouble starts when you begin nearing your "ideal" weight.

At this point you may want to ask yourself, would I prefer to weigh more and look as slim as a model, or be "fatter" and weigh the same as a model? If you're like most people, you'll see that weight is not the be all and end all.

(Some people, in fact, put on weight right at the start even while losing bulk. As long as you're looking and feeling better, it shouldn't be a problem.)

Still, it helps to calculate that ideal weight mentioned above so you have something to aim for when starting out. Traditionally this is done by picking an arbitrary number: "I want to lose a stone" or "I want to get to 11 stone". More recently it might be done by working out your Body Mass Index (BMI) by dividing your weight in kilograms by your height in metres squared. A score between 18.5 and 25 is considered normal; either side of it you're either underweight or overweight; above 30 and you're obese.

But BMI doesn't account for gender or variations in body type, body-fat percentage or fat distribution. A high muscle mass, for instance, would not be taken into account, nor would a measure of visceral fat around the belly, which is more harmful than the fat that sits under the skin.

In time, we at Real Meal Revolution aim to incorporate various measures into the Pie of Life to better determine the end goals for our individual RMR dieters, but for now we make use of two physical variables that offer a somewhat more nuanced guidance than a simple thumbsuck number or BMI measurement.

The first is a more accurate measure of weight, which incorporates both gender and body frame types along with height.

Our chart offers two possible readings: ideal weight and what we call Awesome weight. The former is the weight you might be at peak physical health, calculated using an approved medical table. But the latter, in which we allow for a little leeway, is a weight we prefer to recommend because, while it offers almost all the health benefits of ideal weight, it is more likely to be sustainable and offer you room to live an awesome life without obsessing over your scale. (Note: this method is more accurate than BMI, we feel, though it is still not foolproof, as it doesn't account for age and bone density, for instance.)

The second measurement is a simple waist-hip circumference ratio measurement that is based on the fact that a lower waist-hip ratio is indicative of better health, essentially because you have less fat around the gut; it also means you'll be slimmer and look better in the mirror. In this instance, there is no need to differentiate between an ideal and Awesome ratio: they are the same. (There isn't as much health data on waist circumference as there is on weight loss, but this will likely come in time.)

We believe that aiming for your Awesome weight in conjunction with an Awesome waist-hip ratio gives you a truer and more meaningful way to get to Awesome than a simple measure of weight. Of course, for more accurate (and expensive) measurements you could always see a professional. And in particular you could get your biomarkers for optimum health tested on a regular basis – when they're all spot on, then you're probably at your ideal weight. (See p168.)

Whatever you choose, we recommend you avoid the scale on a daily basis; rather focus on getting to Awesome.

To find your Awesome numbers ...

Use the chart on p172 to find your ideal and Awesome weights.

Use the chart on p174 to find your Awesome hip-waist ratio.

For more on biomarkers see p168.

For a more accurate score, test yourself for Awesomeness by doing the Reality Check test at RealMealRevolution.com.

WORKING OUT YOUR AWESOME TARGETS

First, calculate roughly how much weight you want to lose by subtracting your awesome weight from your current weight.

Second, calculate how long you will spend in Restoration.

Minimum of one week

Additional week for every 10lb (5kg) you want to lose

Maximum of 12 weeks

(There may be minor weight gain in this phase or anything up to 1lb (0.5kg) weight loss per week.)

Round up your answer to the nearest week.

Third, calculate how long you will spend in Transformation:

You will be in Transformation until you reach your Awesome weight.

Expect to lose at least 1-2lb (0.5–1kg) per week – an average of 1½lb (0.75kg).

To calculate how long this will take:

Transformation Weeks = (Current weight – Awesome weight) ÷ 0.75

Round up your answer to the nearest week.

Now copy the chart below and fill in the gaps to start plotting your journey.

In the first row, write down the date you start your week of Observation, your weight and your waist-hip ratio.

Once you have calculated how many weeks you will be spending in each phase, use a calendar and the pounds-per-week guidelines on the previous page to enter your start dates for the following phases and the weight you aim to be on those dates.

My long walk to Awesome!	DATE	WEIGHT	WAIST-HIP RATIO
Start of Observation			
Start of Restoration			
Start of Transformation			
Start of Preservation			

Now stick this on your wall, fridge or on the back of your toilet door. Take it down when you get to your target weight and/or ratio – or simply when you're feeling healthy and good about yourself, and like what you see when you look in the mirror.

Right, let's get to it.

2.4 THE PHASES

2.4.1 OBSERVATION

In any transformation you go through – dietary or otherwise – it is vitally important to know what your starting point is or was. It's easy to get disheartened when you're six months down the line and have forgotten how bad your health or your weight was.

Observation is, as you might imagine, the easiest phase (though it comes with homework) – it is also the most likely to be overlooked.

OBSERVATION ONLY TAKES ONE WEEK BUT IT IS THE MOST CRITICAL WEEK OF THE LOT. WE EMPHASISE: DO IT, AND DO IT PROPERLY.

Unsurprisingly, it's called Observation because it allows you to observe, without changing anything in your life. So, though you are officially on the Real Meal 2.0 programme at this point, you're not actually dieting yet. For the next seven days, continue to eat as per usual. Until you have reached the end of the week don't change your normal eating patterns in any way.

Observation works in two ways. It acts as your rock-bottom snapshot and thus an incredible motivator in the weeks to come, and it serves as a reality check for you. We find that many people don't realise quite how serious their health and lifestyle situation is until the end of this week. Our Observation exercises have been designed to track and report back to you just how bad, or not-that-bad, things really are.

We've got a series of manual tools for you to use in the pages to come, but if you prefer the comprehensive digital route take a look at the tracking tools at RealMealRevolution.com. You can download BANT, our meal tracking app, from the PlayStore or the App Store.

Either way, follow each step here.

OBSERVE
Take a before photograph – in your underwear (if you want to lose more than 1½ stone)

We know, right? But yes.

For a lot of people, taking a before picture in their underwear is one of the hardest things they've ever done. Before (and even after) photos are tough because they reduce us to raw human material. There is literally nowhere to hide – and that's the point. We can't hide behind our personalities or our material goods. A photograph forces us to acknowledge the situation for what it is.

Before you get all cringy, consider two things: first, you're not obliged to share your photo with anyone; and second, whether you're a high-profile big shot or you fly beneath the radar, you're no more or less human than anyone else. Being in your underwear in front of your mobile phone, with only you around, is actually a harmless place to be. You know you're overweight, unhealthy or both. You know you want to change what you see.

The mental side to embracing a new diet is critical to the diet's success – which is why we have spent so much time emphasising the Pie of Life – and this is a genuine moment of truth. If you are too afraid to take your before (and after) photograph, or are dismissive of the idea, there is a real chance that you have not accepted where you are in this process.

Taking the photo will help liberate you.

Now, take off your clothes and take that photo. Pull the plaster. Commit.

Weigh And Measure yourself

We call this the WAM in our group meetings, and it's vitally important (though not as important as the before photograph). Weigh yourself and take your waist measurement (level across your belly button without letting the tape cut into your flesh).

You may have done this before in goal-setting. Do it again. Make it official.

From here on WAM yourself once a week. We suggest doing it on Wednesday – because WAM Wednesday has a ring to it (and is easy to remember).

Track what you eat

Take note of absolutely everything you eat for the entire week: every nut, apple, glass of water, slice of bread, tablespoon of salad dressing, piece of pie, chip, doughnut, soft drink. Everything. This requires work, it's hard and it's irritating, but you absolutely have to do it. Importantly, you have to track the macronutrient ratio, so you'll need an app to do it. Use our free BANT meal tracker app or find something similar online. If you want to keep it old-school, write it all down and ask a health coach or dietitian to break it down for you at the week's end.

Whatever you do, be honest about your consumption. This isn't an insurance health survey. No-one is going to see it unless you show it to them.

Keep an eating journal

Write in your journal before and after you eat. It might sound like overkill, but do it anyway. Give special consideration to what made you hungry. Try to work out if you were genuinely hungry or if there was something else to it: a craving for something to spoil yourself, the temptation of a smell, a moment of procrastination, an emotion that needed satisfying such as emptiness, anger, happiness, frustration. It doesn't need to be Tolstoy. Just a couple of lines per meal or snack.

As an example, your journal might look something like this:

11:00am Mmm, the smell of freshly baked bread. Yum!

11:15am Took that sandwich down like it was nobody's
business.

12:00pm Ashamed of myself. How can I be so powerless to
a stupid piece of bread. It wasn't even sourdough.

Some good tracking apps have a journal function too, so look out for that if you prefer the tech route. The added bonus is it's nice to have all your information consolidated.

Check your bloods

As we've seen, a lot of us follow the RMR diet for health reasons and not necessarily weight loss. You may have signed up after a health scare or seeing a blood result. Either way, taking bloods is something you may want to consider. We strongly recommend getting your blood-pressure and blood-glucose and blood-insulin levels tested, but there is a range of tests to consider. See p168 for more.

Get stuck into the Pie of Life

This is the ideal point to start actively incorporating the ideas from the earlier Pie of Life section into your RMR lifestyle. Turn to p169 and get cracking on the exercises to work out exactly how you're spending your time and how you can better allocate your time from here on.

PUTTING YOUR OBSERVATION TO WORK

At the end of your week of Observation, having done the necessary, you will have a detailed picture of your eating habits. Combine this information with your Pie of Life charts (see p169), and you'll have a complete overview of your health and lifestyle. Review it and take it in. It should tell you who you hang out with, what you do with your time, what you eat and, most importantly, what the health implications of your lifestyle are.

For the most part, just doing the exercise will give you an idea of what you need to change. We recommend trying it in a group environment, preferably with people like you, and sharing your observations if you're confident enough. This can be a particularly instructive process.

File your health data – it will make for an interesting comparison in the weeks and months ahead.

Read over your week of journal entries. Think about the negative entries you entered when you ate badly: snippets like "I regret eating that" or "I'm so bloated". As part of your planning, turn to the end date in your journal and write a week of only positive entries. That will create a mental picture of what you should feel like after you eat. Some examples of positive entries would be "That meal made me feel amazing" or "My mood is stable".

Once your week of observation is complete, you will have a snapshot of yourself at ground zero. If you've done a thorough job and are honest with yourself, you should be able to spot your problem areas without much difficulty. If you'd prefer an expert opinion, take your Pie of Life and Observation results to a health coach, life coach or Certified Banting Coach, and they'll give you more qualified feedback.

With the results in, it's time to start changing things...

2.4.2 RESTORATION

A strict LCHF diet that eliminates carbohydrate intake to almost zero (less than 30g per day) will see you switch to a metabolic state known as ketosis: rather than burning glucose (from carbs) you will be burning ketone bodies (from fat). There is a pronounced adaption process involved and different people are affected differently.

In *The Real Meal Revolution* we recommended to readers to dive straight into ketogenic mode but to be wary of the side effects when they did. These could range from headaches, nausea and crankiness – all standard sugar-withdrawal symptoms – to more concerning side effects such as thinning hair, brittle nails and aggressive flares of gout and gall stones. The poor health that stems from a long-term carb-heavy diet is the root cause of these problems, but the shock to the system of the switch and resulting dramatic weight loss is what brings them on.

There are conflicting opinions on the matter. Go cold turkey – throw away the junk foods immediately, eat nothing but real food, quit gluten and sugar, keep carbs below 30g, up the healthy fat intake – or ease into it?

Both approaches have their pros and cons, but with Real Meal 2.0 we prefer the latter option, only going ketogenic in the third phase, Transformation. While going cold turkey often generates radical weight loss and dramatic improvements in blood readings and overall health, we've noticed from our members' database that a portion of those who dive in hard early reach a plateau or experience side effects. And even before that, the fast approach doesn't allow you the opportunity to establish the strong habits you may need to keep you mentally on track. The fact that slow and consistent weight loss has been shown to be more likely to be sustained is a further consideration.

Prof Noakes took a year before he gave up taking sugar in his tea, and we think he has a point (though we would encourage you to break his record by about 50 weeks).

While acknowledging the slow and steady approach, this isn't to say you won't lose weight during Restoration. This phase is in itself similar to the Paleo diet, and many RMR dieters make significant progress here, with some able to skip Transformation entirely and move directly to Preservation.

REVITALISING YOUR GUT

From a specific physiological point of view, gut health is our prime concern during Restoration. This is because the damage that gluten and a diet rich in inflammatory foods can do is immense, something we are only recently coming to appreciate.

When you reduce your carb intake and start eating real food, your gut will have much better resources to convert into nutrients for your body. You will effectively be getting more (fuel) from less (food), which results in weight loss. But your body will only transform to a level that your gut is able to sustain. In other words, if your gut is not firing on all cylinders, it simply won't be able to process enough nutrients for your body from a small enough quantity of food. This means you would still need to consume more food than you would with a healthy gut in order to supply your body and brain with enough nutrients to signal satiety and nourish your organs, your muscles and your brain. This is, we believe, a likely explanation for many frustrating plateaus.

According to our data, almost half of RMR dieters plateau at some point on their path to a healthy weight. While the state of your gut may well be what's applying the brakes, there are several other possibilities, which we discuss under "Hacks" (see p139).

Beyond that, there are strong correlations between gut health and inflammation throughout the body, and between gut permeability and psychological wellbeing – both are vital for general health.

The broad goals of Restoration are straightforward:
- remove sugar and gluten from your diet, along with all Red-list foods, and
- restore the health of your gut by reintroducing foods that a) fertilise your bowel with beneficial bacteria and food for those bacteria, and b) help your body rebuild your gut lining.

It is a phase that may well yield significant weight-loss results, but don't be concerned if it doesn't; some RMR dieters don't lose weight until Transformation, when total carb intake is significantly reduced.

By the end of Restoration, you should experience some or all of the following:
- weight loss;
- improved, more stable mood;
- ease or disappearance of irritable bowel syndrome, ulcerative colitis, abdominal bloating and other gut and bowel complaints,
- improved focus;
- reduction or disappearance of acne and skin complaints;
- improved sleep.

You may experience a number of other positive effects too.

THE PROCESS
Clear out

Start by overhauling your kitchen (and yourself).

This is another one of those important psychological moments in your mission to turn your health around, a process to allow you to kick things off in the right frame of mind. Head into your kitchen and chuck out everything that contains *any* ingredients on the red list. Don't lie to yourself. There will be foods, drinks and condiments you absolutely love that you think won't make a difference. The passion-fruit cordial, the ketchup, the Worcestershire sauce, the emergency ice cream in the freezer... It must all go in one great symbolic cleansing.

The clear-out is best done on the weekend (at the end of your Observation phase) so you don't have to rush it. If possible get your partner or a friend to help you with the process. A witness adds accountability. Take a photograph of all the unhealthy carbs and processed foods you're piling up before throwing them away – a snapshot that you will return to in the future with amazement.

Read some of the labels of the junk you're binning. Work out how many teaspoons of sugar they contain (1 teaspoon = 4g). Many breakfast cereals are *a quarter added sugar*. Some condiments *are a half added sugar*. Think about how they've contributed to your physique and your health.

This is an act of motivation and practicality. Just doing it will serve as a mental marker, a turning point for you. It also removes any temptation from your house, which will assist in times of weakness in the weeks and months to come.

Stock up

Once you have cleared out, you need to stock up – and be smart about it. (Reminder: don't stock up without clearing out first: that's like building a palace on top of a swamp.)

Run through the staples recipes in the back of the book and go shopping for Green- and Orange-list foods only. Make a homemade ketchup (easy) and mayo (easier than you think), and all the rest.

When you cut out sugar, you're going to want to eat everything in sight, so make sure you've got a supply of healthy snacks, like biltong, hard cheese, roast chicken, boiled eggs, olives, cherry tomatoes, celery, cucumber and (healthy) dips and pâtés. You need to make sure you are ready for every possible scenario, so keep a supply of food in your car and your office as well to prepare for untimely hunger pangs.

Go on Red alert

Cut the entire Red and Light-Red lists from your diet. Most importantly, avoid foods containing any form of sugar or gluten, without exception. There are no limits to how much you eat as long as it's from the Green and Orange lists. Your carb intake will naturally drop without the Red-list foods, but real low-carb eating will come in the next phase.

Keep WAMming yourself

Don't forget WAM Wednesday: weigh and measure yourself once a week.

114

Embrace healthy fats

Eat healthy fats. Make friends with them. Realise that not only are they good for you, but they will also naturally inhibit your temptation to binge. You'll find plenty of them on the Green list.

Keep observing

Keep writing in your journal and updating your lifestyle tables. Once a week is fine at this point – just make sure you do it because it will reveal how subtle changes to your diet show up in your lifestyle and how changes to your diet and lifestyle show up in your psyche and your emotions.

Fertilise your gut

We like to talk about fertilising your gut – because when you're looking after your gut biome that's pretty much what you're doing. You're giving it the right foods to let the gut flora down there grow and thrive and ultimately work to your benefit. Given that your gut is about the size of a tennis court – as we saw earlier – and it's where all the action happens, you may want to consider it Wimbledon Centre Court. You're about to play the game of your life, so best to prepare (repair) it well. Water it, fertilise it, look after it.

There are two types of fertiliser to help regenerate your gut health:

- *Bone broth:* rich with all the nutrients and minerals your body needs to rebuild the intestinal linings (and any other tissue).
- *Fermented foods and drinks:* rich with nutrients as a result of the fermentation process; foods like natural yoghurt, sauerkraut

and kimchi and drinks like kefir and kombucha help repopulate the gut biome with healthy bacteria or feed the bacteria that are already there.

FERMENTED FOODS v PROBIOTICS

There have been few clinical trials on the effects of fermentation foods on gut health – the financing of such trials is tricky, we imagine – but the anecdotal evidence for positive effects is compelling. Consuming fermented drinks and foods has been widely reported (for centuries) to be of benefit and is advocated by doctors and health specialists globally. The assumed reasoning is that bacteria in the fermented foods help rejuvenate bacteria populations in the gut, but the extent to which these foods actually repopulate the gut biome has not been established. Our networked LCHF experts who advocate fermented foods for gut health don't offer much more than "introduce fermented foods to your diet". So our prescriptions are only guidelines. Listen to your body and see what works for you.

On a related note, taking probiotics pills or drinking probiotics liquids is thought to be less effective than actually eating probiotic foods (foods rich in bacteria as a result of fermentation), for a variety of reasons. While there is preliminary research showing that certain probiotics may treat specific diseases, the idea of probiotic supplements being a cure-all is a long way from acceptance. Many specialists, such as Alessio Fasano, mentioned earlier, acknowledge the promise of probiotics but advise against taking them on a daily basis. Fasano says "absolutely no" to a daily prescription, though he does advocate a diet rich in probiotic foods for those with poor gut health. See p206.

We suggest easing yourself gently into gut rejuvenation, spending the first two or three weeks of Restoration prepping and researching. Perhaps spend a few hours on the weekend making broth, kimchi or sauerkraut. (The longest any of these foods should take you to make is two weeks.) If you're not going to make all your own probiotic foods, track down where you can buy them. Work out what you like the look of and what you think will work for you.

Once your probiotic foods and drinks are ready, and you're feeling comfortable without sugar and gluten in your diet (and you haven't cheated!), introduce your fertilisers. You could, of course, buy them on day one and start immediately, but bear in mind that, being live foods, they are difficult to store for long periods and can be expensive. If you go this route, don't overdo things.

We recommend one portion of either a broth or a fermented food every day; the latter can be either a half of cup of a fermented drink or a tablespoon of fermented vegetables. It will be a bit weird to start. But once you've done it for a day or two, it will grow on you and you should start craving it.

For more on Restoration foods and recipes see *The Restoration Station* on p190 and the meal plans that follow.

HOW LONG DOES RESTORATION LAST?

Minimum of 1 week

Extra week for every extra 10lb (5kg) you need to lose

Maximum of 12 weeks

HOW MUCH FAT CAN I EAT DURING RESTORATION?

At this point you can welcome fat back into your life. You're not trying to lose weight yet. You are cleansing yourself of junk and you'll need to feel full and enriched. As a rough guide, eat one to two thumbs of healthy fat per meal (bearing in mind a snack isn't a meal).

For more on fermented foods and gut health...

■ Read "Fermented foods, microbiota, and mental health: ancient practice meets nutritional psychiatry" by Eva Selhub, Alan Logan and Alison Bested from *Journal of Physiological Anthropology* (2014), available at www.ncbi.nlm.nih.gov.

2.4.3 TRANSFORMATION

You're now down to the crunch, Transformation, when you can act with decisiveness and start shedding pounds. This phase is effectively the original strict RMR diet, with some important tweaks. It is, as the name suggests, where the major change occurs. You *will* lose weight and improve your health during Transformation – but you need to maintain discipline to do so.

By now you may or may not have lost some weight. More importantly, you will have established healthy eating habits and your gut will be in much better shape, its lining on the mend and microbiome in superior nick. This means you should now have an efficient nutrient-processing machine inside you, requiring less food to extract your body's requirements, with your appetite working in sync with your metabolism.

With the groundwork laid, it's time to severely restrict your carb intake. As outlined earlier in the book, this is the stage where you you reduce the amount of glucose entering your blood and thus reduce the amount of insulin that needs to be produced, which will allow your body to make use of your body fat for fuel. In other words, by dropping your carbs, your body burns fat. (Just note the *How much fat can I eat?* section on p121.)

THE PROCESS
30 or less
Drop your carbohydrate intake to 30 grams per day. In *The Real Meal Revolution* we used 25 grams per day as a guide; this slight tweak is based on recent consultation with experts in the US. In

reality the carbohydrate intake that allows the switch to ketosis varies from individual to individual.

You will need to track this on a meal tracker for accurate results – but as you will have been tracking your meals for at least two weeks, you should have a clear idea of what foods drive up your carb count and thus need to be avoided in this stage.

Green (and Orange) light

Eat food from the Green and Orange A lists only, obeying the limits laid out in the latter. If possible, avoid Orange A entirely.

Keep the Green clean

Continue fertilising with bone broth, kefirs and/or fermented foods, with the exception of kombucha and yoghurt, which are higher in sugar/carbs and now fall on the Orange B list.

Keep track

Track your meals every second week. This is a must-do during Transformation. No matter how much you may or may not know about carb counting and macronutrient ratios, you must track what you eat at this point so you can plot your progress. It's a pain, but it's temporary and necessary. You are only one mouthful away from breaking your carb threshold for the day so track closely! We track every second week because, as we've noted, this is a learning exercise. Eventually you will stop tracking; in the meantime, consider the meal tracker your bike stabilisers.

Also don't forget WAM Wednesday: keep weighing and measuring yourself once a week.

Consider fasting

Skipping meals or several meals in a row is an excellent way to add punch to your "shedding" period because fasting produces excellent fat-burning results. We therefore recommend regular fasting during Transformation, especially if you've hit a stubborn plateau – but only if you're up for it. It can be difficult to get your head around the concept of fasting at first, so avoid it if you think it will make life even tougher or perhaps save it for a halfway-mark upgrade. See p132 for a more detailed overview.

HOW MUCH FAT CAN I EAT DURING TRANSFORMATION?

No more than one thumb of fat (solid or liquid) per meal. Remember, you want to burn your body fat during this phase.

HOW LONG DOES IT TAKE?

We've considered this in *Getting To Awesome* already, but as a reminder: allocate two weeks for every 2 pounds you're aiming to lose. You should lose between 1 and 2 pounds per week during this phase, but don't be surprised if it's more. Some RMR dieters, especially men, have lost up to 1½ stone in a week, though those are the outliers.

Note, however, that you are likely to lose more weight in the middle of Transformation than you will in the beginning or towards the end of it. From our data, it would appear that RMR dieters' bodies take time to become adapted to burning fat before rapid weight loss can occur. Once this is started, the bulk of your weight loss should occur within three months; we've seen some people losing up to 4½ stone in that time, though we usually don't recommend losing too much weight too quickly.

After the period of rapid weight loss is over, those stubborn last few pounds can take some time to shift – be patient.

This is the path you will have to stay on until you reach your Awesome weight. You may be tempted to take your foot off the pedal as you're closing in on it, but that is when you will need to push yourself the most – it's best to keep off the carbs until you're past the chequered flag.

REMEMBER:
KEEP FIGHTING THE GOOD FIGHT

Losing a load of weight and revitalising your health is no mean goal. Keep reminding yourself of this. You will be tempted to quit, probably on a daily or even hourly basis to start. This will get better as you start seeing results – then one day you may have a desperate urge to relapse. Don't.

Be practical. Put less food on your plate. Eat off smaller plates. Say no. Eat slowly and chew your food. Skip meals when you can. Say no again. (See p142 for more practical checklists.)

Make your eating plan work for you rather than letting it dictate your life. If something's not working for you, adapt it. Don't blame your mistakes on anyone but yourself. Decide to win and stop at nothing until you do.

THE REALISATION

By the time you reach your Aweomse weight, you will start finding you no longer feel hungry between meals, and the desire to poke about the fridge and kitchen cupboards at random intervals during the day has disappeared. This is because your body has adapted itself to burning fat and you have regained control over your hunger. As a result you have regained control over food: you no longer allow it to define who you are. You are transformed, both physically and mentally.

This is an epic realisation.

Well done. You've made it. Now you just have to stay like this forever.

2.4.4 PRESERVATION

The hard part is over. Now the most important part: preserving the new status quo.

Because fat is so energy-rich and real foods are so nutritious, by the time you reach Preservation you'll find yourself naturally eating less at meals and throughout the day. Certainly, you'll have cut down on the snacking, and you may find yourself skipping entire meals and barely noticing. This is perfectly fine, and there's no need to feel guilty because you missed breakfast, supposedly the most important meal of the day (NB: it isn't: what you eat or don't eat at any meal is important) or lunch or both. In fact, missing meals by consciously fasting is an excellent way to lower your blood-insulin levels and manage your weight – see p126.

As long as you're healthy and your weight is stable, you can let yourself be guided by your hunger – and the forever rules.

HOW MUCH FAT CAN I EAT DURING PRESERVATION?

Judge this according to your own energy levels. To enter the Preservation phase, you will have lost a significant supply of your body's fat during Restoration and/or Transformation. You'll now need to consume a bit more fat to fuel yourself. Some RMR dieters report consuming up to 300g of fat per day as a helpful guideline, while others are fine without any major change to their fat intake; it depends on satiety and preference.

THE FOREVER RULES
Follow the lists

Follow the Preservation lists.

- Green is, as always, great: eat freely (to hunger).
- Orange is fine but be wary.
- Light-Red may be okay for some people, depending on individual carb thresholds, but be particularly wary and monitor the effects.
- Red is, as always, ruinous: avoid at all costs – and if you stray, realise that you will probably have to respond with a health kick.
- Grey is for you to decide.

For all colours, listen to your body, note how it reacts and respond accordingly.

Keep fertilising

We're seeing the tip of the iceberg when it comes to learning about the gut biome. From our reading, the scientists seem confident that an important part of our medical future lies in this direction, so be sure to keep your gut in fine working order. You want it firing on all cylinders, absorbing nutrients efficiently and preventing toxins from slipping into your bloodstream.

Drink broth. Eat yoghurt. Make fermented foods and drinks a part of your diet at least twice a week or as often as possible. You'll find yourself naturally eating more and more fermented foods as time goes by.

Fast often

Finally, consider the benefits of fasting to help maintain your Awesome weight or to get back on track if you've slipped. We recommend to all RMR dieters (except those mentioned in *Who should not fast?* on p138) that they fast on a regular basis, if only a 16-hour fast once a week – which is barely one missed breakfast. Once your body has settled into its more satiated, fat-burning state, it is easier than you'd imagine. In time you'll be able to do it without thinking about it. See p132 for more.

WHAT IF YOU SLIP?

React quickly and effectively. If you enjoy fasting, fast. Alternatively, go back to basics. We suggest three days of Transformation eating in combination with a 16:8 fast for every cheat meal.

If you fall off the wagon completely, head all the way back to Observation and follow the steps again from your current state. If you've done it once you can do it again... See p160.

2.4.5 SUMMARY

Give or take a little detail, you may say that Real Meal 2.0 has two levels of strictness. After the one-off week of Observation, a lighter form of RMR dieting – the Restoration and Preservation phases – bookends the really serious weight-loss stage of Transformation. Those details are important, of course (and Observation is critical, don't forget), but this is broadly accurate.

There is a chance, if you're not particularly insulin resistant, that you may spend little or even no time in Transformation – which is wonderful. Similarly, if you're very insulin resistant (most likely diabetic or pre-diabetic), you probably shouldn't ever leave Transformation – in which case it effectively becomes your Transformation *and* Preservation phase. If you've lost plenty of weight and your blood work is looking a whole lot better, then you will no doubt agree it's worth the effort.

Wherever you lie on the spectrum, you'll need to preserve according to your own reactions while continuously listening to your body.

Here are the phases in short:

OBSERVATION

1. Snapshot – take a before photo (if you want to lose more than 1½ stone).
2. WAM – weigh and measure yourself.
3. Bloods – consider getting your blood work done, specifically measuring your blood-glucose and blood-insulin levels.
4. Don't change – eat as usual for a week.
5. Keep track – record everything you eat, being sure to measure your macronutrient intake.

6. Start a food journal – and write in it regularly.

7. Review – go through the journal and your resulting dietary-lifestyle snapshot at week's end.

RESTORATION

1. Clear out – conduct a full clear-out of your kitchen, getting rid of all Red-list foods.

2. Stock up – do the big shop for the right ingredients, and cook some delicious kitchen staples.

3. Red alert – remove the entire Red list from your life.

4. No limits – don't stress about how much you eat.

5. Healthy fats – eat healthy fats (in which case you will naturally eat less).

6. Observe – write in your journal and fill in your Pie Charts of Life once a week.

7. Fertilise your gut – one dose of fertiliser per day.

8. WAM Wednesday – weigh and measure yourself.

TRANSFORMATION

1. 30g or less – reduce your carbohydrate intake to 30 grams per day.

2. Green light – eat from the Green list and stick to the limits on Orange A.

3. Keep fertilising – continue fertilising with bone broth and/or fermented foods on a daily basis.

4. WAM Wednesday – weigh and measure yourself.

5. Keep track – track everything that passes your lips.

PRESERVATION

1. Follow the lists – Green: eat freely (to hunger); Orange: eat occasionally; Light-Red: enjoy according to your carb threshold; Red: avoid at all costs; Grey: your call.

2. Keep fertilising – continue fertilising with bone broth, yoghurts and/ or fermented foods on a daily basis.

3. Fast often – fast according to your preferences and requirements.

4. Three days of Transformation with 16:8 fasting for every cheat meal.

FAT CONSUMPTION SUMMARY:

RESTORATION	TRANSFORMATION	PRESERVATION
Get used to eating fat	Burn excess body fat	Sustain new physique on fat
As much as you're comfortable with	No more than 1 thumb of fat per meal (liquid or solid)	Depends on satiety and preference

PART 3

HACKS, FAQs & OTHER RESOURCES

3.1 HACKS

Tips, tactics and ideas to solve your health and weight-loss problems:

3.1.1 Intermittent Fasting

3.1.2 Breaking Through The Plateau

3.1.3 The Awesome Checklist

3.1.4 Problem Food (And Drink)

3.2 FAQs

Our most frequently asked questions

3.3 OTHER RESOURCES

Tests, charts and the experts behind the science

3.3.1 Your Insulin Resistance And General Health

3.3.2 Your Pie Charts of Life

3.3.3 Your Awesome Charts

3.3.4 The Experts

3.1 HACKS

In online lingo, a life hack is a clever way to solve a tricky problem. Losing weight, becoming healthy and getting to Awesome can certainly present a few tricky problems, so here are our lifestyle hacks to keep the journey moving.

3.1.1 INTERMITTENT FASTING

Intermittent fasting is a lifestyle hack to encourage weight loss and related good health or maintain a consistent weight, and it's so effective we consider it a critical addition to the Real Meal 2.0 armoury. It can be wielded with great effect to give added punch to your weight loss during Transformation, and we recommend it as a long-term strategy in Preservation. But it can take a little getting used to, both physically and mentally, and it needs to be done right for good results.

THE BACKGROUND

If you grew up being told breakfast was the most important meal of the day and should never be missed, you may hesitate at the idea of fasting. And if you've ever been advised to snack regularly and stick to a strict meal plan – possibly including "mid-meals" – it may sound like heresy. It's not.

In days gone by, most of our ancestors ate only one meal a day without a problem, and it was unusual to "break the fast" in the morning. Ready access to cheap food has made eating a more regular occurrence, encouraged by Big Food manufacturers who not only push the idea that breakfast is the most important meal of the day but also that you should include their high-carbohydrate, high-sugar cereals in yours...

Give it a second's thought and fasting makes perfect sense. You eat less food. Simple.

More than that, however, it significantly reduces your insulin levels, which encourages fat burning and a range of related health benefits.

Every time you eat, your body produces insulin; the longer you don't eat, the more time your insulin levels have to drop. Fasting has been shown to dramatically accelerate weight loss, increase metabolism and mental focus, and reduce the symptoms of, and in some cases reverse, type-2 diabetes.

For those who are severely insulin resistant and who may take 10 or 12 hours to use up their glycogen stores, fasting can be the tactic that finally sees them lower their insulin levels sufficiently to get into the fat-burning state and break a weight-loss plateau. It is also effective for those who aren't following strict low-carb diets.

On a related note, athletes with ketogenic metabolisms, especially long-distance and ultra-marathon runners, often perform at their best when they don't take in any sustenance (apart from water) for the entire duration of an event.

WHAT ARE THE BENEFITS OF FASTING?

Lower blood-sugar and insulin levels

Weight loss

Weight-loss plateau breaker

More energy

Improved digestion

Improved concentration

Reduced chronic inflammation

Possible cell-regeneration and anti-ageing effects

Convenient and inexpensive

The basic advice

1. Don't be scared of missing meals. There is a liberating element to fasting: you don't have to prepare and eat a meal! Spend an extra 20 minutes in bed before going to work, skip lunch and go for a walk, work through lunch and leave early...

2. But if you fast, best do it right. In which case, read on.

What can you eat or drink during a fast?

The point of a fast is to prevent the body from producing insulin, so eating is out. Discipline is essential for it to be effective.

Water, tea, herbal teas and coffee are all fine and are in fact encouraged, especially to start, to get through the hunger pangs. But your tea and coffee must be black (and sugar- and sweetener-free). Bone broth is also recommended, especially during longer fasts, to replenish lost vitamins, minerals and salts (see p193).

What are the various fast durations?

Many ascetics have been known to fast for weeks or even months at a time – but relax, this isn't what we have in mind for you...

A beginner should fast for a minimum of 12, preferably 16 hours, to allow insulin levels to drop sufficiently to encourage fat-burning.

We suggest using one or more of four general fast durations. The first three are recommended by the Canadian low-carb advocate Jason Fung, and the fourth by the BBC's well-known Michael Mosley (see references on p138).

16:8 FAST Fast for 16 hours and eat in the eight-hour window that follows.
This is easier than it sounds because the 16 hours also includes sleep. Effectively it means skipping breakfast and only eating two meals in a day. Can be done daily or as needed.

24-HOUR FAST Fast for 24 hours.
This would usually be from dinner until dinner, which means skipping two meals in a row. Can be done up to three times a week.

36-HOUR FAST Fast for 36 hours.
This fast usually incorporates two nights of sleep and a complete day without food. Use it once or, at most, twice a week.

5:2 FAST Eat normally for five days of the week, and fast for any two days of the week.

This is a longer-term regimen as recommended by Michael Mosley, who was so impressed by what he learned while researching and filming a television series on food that he developed and popularised the so-called 5:2 diet. It advises a severely reduced calorie intake on fasting days; as such, it's not strictly a fast and not necessarily low-carb, though we would recommend carb restrictions on those days.

Which fasting method is right for you?

Longer fasting methods generally work best for people with severe insulin resistance. If you are a type-2 diabetic, or pre-diabetic, you could consider up to three 24-hour fasts a week with the occasional 36-hour fast. On other days you could use the 16:8 fast.

Shorter fasts are usually sufficient for those who don't have a lot of weight to lose and for maintenance.

During which RMR diet phases should you fast?

From Restoration onwards you could fast whenever you are comfortable managing it in your lifestyle and feel you need the extra boost. It's recommended particularly in Transformation to encourage an extra bout of fat burning, and regularly in Preservation as a maintenance strategy.

How do you get started?

Slowly. At first, fasting can be both a physiological and mental challenge as your body and mind adapt. In time, the hunger pangs become much easier to handle and often go unnoticed. Kick off with a 16:8 fast and see how your body responds to it.

Some people find that once their fast is over they want to eat everything in sight, which obviously isn't ideal. For your meals during this time make sure that you are eating enough fat to sustain you through the periods when you aren't eating.

Once you've mastered the 16:8 fast, you can try fasting for longer periods of time as you prefer or need.

How do you break a fast?

Without overeating.

One of the temptations of intermittent fasting, especially when you're starting out, is gorging when you're done or "rewarding" yourself with poor food choices. In which case you're doing it wrong and it rather defeats the object...

Don't use fasting – whether planned or unplanned – as an excuse to binge. Be prepared and keep a healthy snack on stand-by in case of emergency. We recommend breaking a fast with a bowl of broth, a handful of nuts or a piece of cheese half an hour before your next meal; enough time for your snack to digest and prevent overeating.

Should you develop a fasting routine?

While it may be a good idea to break your fasts in a similar way each time to prevent overeating, we advise against developing a regular fasting routine.

One of the apparent risks of fasting every day is that your body can eventually adapt to this strategy by lowering your metabolism, the opposite of what you want it to do. To prevent this we recommend fasting randomly and out of sequence to keep the body guessing.

What are the potential side effects of fasting?

Dehydration. A lack of salt and too much caffeine can cause dehydration. Drink enough non-caffeinated fluids to stay hydrated, and ensure you have enough salt, especially during long fasts.

Headaches. A by-product of dehydration.

Muscle cramps. Another potential problem due to dehydration and shortage of salt. Bone broth with added salt is a good remedy if this is affecting you.

Constipation. Yet another problem potentially exacerbated by dehydration. Avoid this while not fasting by upping your fibre and ensuring you're eating vegetables with the skins still on, along with the Real Meal essentials: green leafy vegetables and healthy fats such as avocados, seeds and nuts.

Who should NOT fast?

Intermittent fasting is not recommended for infants, growing children, pregnant/breastfeeding moms or anyone who suffers from a medical condition or is taking chronic medication that may be adversely affected by skipping meals.

For more on fasting...

We recommend looking into the work of Jason Fung. His first book, *The Obesity Code* (Greystone, 2016), gives a good introduction to fasting, while his most recent, *The Complete Guide To Fasting* (with Jimmy Moore; Victory Belt Publishing, 2016), is dedicated entirely to the topic; the subtitle is *Heal your body through intermittent, alternate-day, and extended fasting.* For more on the 5:2 diet, see *The Fast Diet: Lose weight, stay healthy, live longer* by Michael Mosley and Mimi Spencer (Short Books, 2014).

3.1.2 BREAKING THROUGH THE PLATEAU

A frequently encountered frustration when following a weight-loss programme is the dreaded plateau. Things seemed to be going so well, the weight was coming off – then all of a sudden the pounds stopped shifting. You've made no progress in two weeks and now you don't know what to do.

Chill. Many have hit this barrier before you and you've got lots of options to consider.

First, exclude the obvious reasons – the diet-troubleshooting equivalent of checking that your computer is plugged in and turned on:

Have you slipped without noticing?

Honestly review your eating habits since you hit the plateau. Are you following the guidelines closely or have you quietly fallen back into old habits because things were going so well?

Has there been an upheaval or change of routine in your life?

Any possible life stressors can affect cortisol and thus insulin levels. A major event, such as a death in the family or loss of a job, would be a more obvious culprit, but even something apparently minor may set you back. Have you or your partner been travelling? Have your children been sick? Have you been working long hours on deadline? Are there other possible disturbances to your hormonal balance that need to be resolved?

Is your gut health up to scratch?

This potential reason for decelerating weight loss may be less obvious than the first two, but it's worth considering. Though it's difficult to quantify just how important this factor may be in overcoming weight plateaus, we believe that an insufficiently healed gut is frequently the culprit.

The thinking is this: if your gut biome is significantly out of balance – due to poor eating habits in the past, overuse of antibiotics, and so on – your gut lining won't be able to process nutrients from the food you eat efficiently enough to maintain weight loss. In other words, you will have to eat too much food to get the right amount of nutrients into your bloodstream. And, as previously discussed, the relatively poor state of your gut will have other knock-on effects, encouraging inflammation and keeping your appestat from operating efficiently. In such an instance, you could be both malnourished *and* hungry...

You may think this is odd, especially if you've lost a load of weight already, but early weight loss occurs easily in Transformation because of your lowered insulin levels, gut health notwithstanding. It's after that effect has played itself out that a damaged gut can hold you back.

The implications of this theory are far-reaching. First, it means your gut didn't heal itself as it should have during Restoration. If it had, your weight-loss journey would proceed in a smoother and more predictable manner from the day you significantly drop your carbs. Second, it shows just how sensitive your gut is to cheating, especially if that cheat contains wheat. The bottom line: if you heal your gut upfront, your weight-loss journey is more likely to be unhindered from the day you significantly drop your carb intake.

Consider spending a rigorous session – two weeks or more – in Restoration to repair your gut.

WHAT NEXT?

If you're confident your plateau isn't being caused by any of the likely suspects above, then we recommend running a full diagnostic check on the status of your diet. That means completing the Awesome checklist...

3.1.3 THE AWESOME CHECKLIST

As we've seen, there's no one-size-fits-all fix for weight loss. We respond to different foods in different ways, and there are a host of variables, both lifestyle- and diet-related, that can affect the way our bodies hold on to our fat stores.

To help keep you on the Getting To Awesome track, we've devised an extended checklist of tips and guidelines that you could be ticking off to overcome a weight plateau (assuming it's not one of the more obvious reasons, as just discussed), or simply make your journey easier. Some may be particularly beneficial to you; others less so. Some have been discussed in detail already; others are hacks we've come across that we've found to be particularly effective.

The most likely non-dietary suspects – which also affect your levels of motivation and the general joy you get out of life – that could be influencing your health and weight are:

- **Exercise and physical health.** Are you exercising as much and as effectively as possible?
- **Sleep.** Are you sleeping well and feeling energised during the day?
- **Stress.** Are you actively dealing with your life stresses and getting the balance right between work and play, socialising and me-time, and general wellbeing?
- **Goal-keeping.** Have you set achievable goals and are you staying focused on them?

And then, of course, there is the most obvious factor:

■ **Diet.** Are you eating the right things in the right ways?

You may do perfectly well without following some of the recommendations starting over the page, or even many of them, but if you are struggling at any point while following the RMR diet then go through the list one by one to discover if you've been neglecting a critical area or simply overlooking something minor that could make a big difference.

Any box you honestly cannot tick is something that will probably get you closer to Awesome.

Note: if you continue to hold on to the weight after being in Transformation for a month, and have ticked all the boxes, consider seeking medical attention. Check with your doctor whether any medication you're taking – be it prescribed or not – may be affecting your weight and, if so, whether there is an alternative option (that won't compromise your health). Consider monitoring your cortisol, adrenal hormones, vitamin D-3, B12 or thyroid hormone, which may have an effect on weight loss.

For physical wellbeing, am I –

☐ Following an enjoyable and sensible exercise regimen, with workouts and activities that I look forward to and are sustainable in the long run?

☐ Doing one to three high-intensity workouts a week?

☐ Exercising regularly with a partner or attending group workouts or facilitated training sessions where I will be held accountable?

☐ Carrying a spare gym bag to the office or in my car?

☐ Not eating before exercise, and preferably exercising in a fasted state? (Exercise after 16 hours or more of fasting – then break your fast with broth afterwards.)

☐ Preparing for a physical goal, or event that I have paid for and am doing with friends? (So you can't back out.)

☐ Stretching once a day?

☐ Resting with no exercise for at least one full day per week?

☐ Taking the stairs rather than the lift? (Try to do it for any trip of three storeys or less.)

☐ Switching between standing and sitting at my desk or workplace?

☐ Spending 20 minutes of my lunch break or some part of the day walking around outside?

To get the most from my sleep or help me sleep better, am I –

☐ Getting 7-9 hours of quality sleep per night?

☐ Avoiding caffeine after lunch?

☐ Limiting alcohol intake?

☐ Avoiding sleeping pills? (Unless prescribed by your doctor.)

☐ Avoiding exercise too late in the day?

☐ Avoiding digital screens for at least two hours before I go to bed? (Set your devices to switch to Night Shift after 7pm.)

☐ Spending time before bed actively winding down and clearing my mind? In whatever way works:
- listening to relaxing music,
- thinking about the day gone by, and practising positive thoughts for the day to come,
- meditating/praying,
- drinking a warm drink such as almond milk or chai tea,
- having a bath,
- lighting candles.

☐ Keeping the lights dim before I go to sleep?

☐ Keeping my bedroom free of electronics? (Turn off your phone and keep it off your bedside table if possible; buy an old-fashioned alarm clock if needs be.)

☐ Reading a real book or magazine in bed?

☐ Sleeping in as dark and as quiet a room as possible?

☐ Sleeping in a room at the optimum temprature (15-19°C)?

☐ Turning on the light and reading when I can't sleep in the middle of the night? (Rather than rolling over and over.)

☐ Taking reenergising naps during the day when necessary?

To best manage my stress, am I –

☐ Teamed up with a friend or partner who is at a similar health and fitness level, with similar weight goals?

☐ Spending time with people who make me feel great, especially people who believe in my goals?

☐ Spending time with friends who like exercising or eating healthily?

☐ Spending less time in situations with friends who encourage me not to look after myself? (See those friends for a morning coffee or afternoon walk, when possible, rather than an evening drink; rather than cutting them off, look to turn negative influences into positive ones.)

☐ Attending a support group of people doing what I'm doing?

☐ Consulting a mentor who has done it before?

☐ Helping someone else with their journey?

☐ Doing things that make me laugh as often as possible?

☐ Meditating, praying or spending time looking at nature for at least ten minutes every day?

☐ Getting a weekly massage or spa treatment – whether paid for or not?

☐ Letting the frustration flow over me and dealing with issues head on, rather than letting them boil on inside me?

☐ Screaming as loudly and hard as I can when I want to explode with stress? (Try doing it underwater.)

☐ Playing a sport such as squash or golf that allows me to smack a ball – and release some frustration! – as hard as I can?

☐ Spending at least two hours a week in nature?

☐ Reminding myself that I am awesome without being thin, and that being awesome is way more important than anything else?

To keep my goals on track, am I –

☐ Keeping a "Before" photo – and looking at it when needed – to remind me of the way I was?

☐ Visualising myself as already slim and healthy? (Picture your face stuck on a picture of the body you want.)

☐ Regularly repeating the SMART goals that I have written down?

☐ Regularly affirming to myself why my goal is important to me and who is counting on me to achieve it?

☐ Setting short-term weekly goals to break down my long-term goal into manageable chunks, and taking each day one at a time?

☐ Focusing on following the RMR diet rules rather than "losing weight"? (Because short-term goals should be about eating the right foods, not losing so many pounds.)

☐ Thinking only about the next pound? (When you're thinking in pounds.)

☐ Rewarding myself – with things that aren't food-related – when I achieve a milestone?

☐ Writing in my journal after eating both good meals and bad meals, and paying attention to how I feel?

☐ Listing all of the foods I crave and reading the list regularly to become unaffected by them?

☐ Keeping my "thin jeans" somewhere I can see them often so I am motivated to wear them again – because I know that I can?

When I eat and drink, am I –

☐ Eating only real, hand-prepared food?

☐ Restricting my carbs to no more than 30g per day?

☐ Eating according to my ideal ratio of fats, proteins and carbs?

☐ Maintaining my gut health by eating fermented foods regularly?

☐ Taking my time when I eat, allowing my satiety hormones to kick in, rather than wolfing my meals?

☐ Sitting down to eat, even when I snack?

☐ Avoiding snacks as much as possible?

147

☐ Refraining from picking when I prepare meals?

☐ Chewing each mouthful ten or more times to slow down and make my food easier to digest?

☐ Taking two teaspoons of apple cider vinegar before meals to lower my glycaemic load?

☐ Tracking everything I eat on a meal tracker? (Temporarily limit your meal variety, if you like, so that it's easier to track what you eat.)

☐ Drinking a glass of water before every meal? (To prevent overeating.)

☐ Watching my alcohol? (Cutting consumption or avoiding it altogether when possible, otherwise choosing whisky and water/soda instead of beer and wine.)

☐ Drinking my coffee and tea black? (Or switch to herbal.)

☐ Eating off a smaller plate to help me control my portion sizes?

☐ Avoiding second helpings to learn what kind of portion sizes I should be eating?

☐ Leaving a mouthful of food behind on my plate to practise conquering my meals rather than allowing them to conquer me?

☐ Fasting according to the 16:8 rule?

☐ Fasting 24 hours straight? (No more than two to three times a week.)

☐ Occasionally fasting for 36 hours? (No more than once a week.)

☐ Breaking my fast with bone broth or a handful of nuts and then only eating again 20 minutes after that?

☐ Brushing my teeth after dinner? (To put a mental full stop on your eating for the day – because so much to do with weight loss is governed by the mind.)

3.1.4 PROBLEM FOOD (AND DRINK)

Throughout Real Meal 2.0 we encourage you to follow your body's cues to work out what dietary details affect you most dramatically. Certain foods are always considered negative, though the sensitivity varies from individual to individual; for instance, sugar, refined carbohydrates and gluten affect different people with varying degrees of toxicity (and with no redeeming health benefits).

Other foods may have some positive attributes and some negative. It's up to you to work out the specifics, with the three categories below deserving special mention.

DAIRY

Dairy has always been a bit of a troublemaker. Some diets, such as Paleo, reject it outright, but the RMR diet generally embraces dairy because of its many potential positives. For example, one cup of milk contains about a quarter of your daily needs of calcium, phosphorous and vitamins D and B2 (riboflavin), as well as significant quantities of vitamin B12 and potassium.

The dairy endorsement does, however, come with a qualification: certain people must steer clear.

Dairy products have long been a complicated and controversial subject for dietitians. From an evolutionary perspective, cow's milk is genetically designed for calves, not for humans, and lactose intolerance is a common condition. But geneticists have shown how some populations in Europe developed an ability to break down lactose and benefit from the nutrients in milk.

For those genetically adapted to drinking milk, go for it. But if you suffer from rashes, hives, bloating, constipation, asthma and other typical allergic responses to milk, then it's best avoided.

But there's more to dairy than milk. When acted on by fungi and bacteria through fermentation, lactose and various other complex proteins that are so bothersome to some are broken down into far more accessible food nutrients that can be highly beneficial to your gut health, as well as providing excellent nutrition. Moreover, the resulting foods can enrich your diet and enjoyment of food enormously.

We recommend avoiding commercial dairy products that are either highly processed (the heat of pasteurisation, for example, kills both good and bad bacteria) or derived from milk from grain-fed cows. These cautions aside, the general rule for dairy products is that the longer they are matured, the more LCHF-appropriate they become. So a commercial yoghurt is still fairly high in carbs and should be eaten sparingly, especially during Transformation. Other products on RMR's Orange list include milk and cottage, cream and soft cheeses, whereas harder cheeses, such as parmigiano and pecorino, are on the Green list.

In summary, different people will react differently to dairy and should therefore monitor how they are affected. If you're unsure, stay away from dairy during Transformation. And if you're struggling to lose weight or break through a plateau, or if you suspect you may be lactose intolerant, forgo dairy entirely and monitor the effects.

THE "DEADLY" NIGHTSHADES
Tomatoes, potatoes, peppers, aubergine

You may have heard of nightshade plants, but did you know they belong to the *Solanaceae* family, which includes tomatoes, tomatillos, potatoes (not sweet potatoes), peppers (chilli, paprika, cayenne pepper and sweet bell peppers) and aubergine?

You'll see them on the Real Meal 2.0 lists where previously they got no mention. This is because anecdotal evidence shows symptoms of nightshade sensitivity to include, among other things, muscle pain and tightness, morning stiffness, poor healing, arthritis, insomnia, gall-bladder problems, heartburn, constipation, headaches, nausea, bloating, flatulence, IBS, poor food absorption and osteoporosis. You might imagine some of those symptoms after a night of serious chilli consumption, but from a potato? A tomato? Apparently, yes.

All living things on the planet have some sort of defence mechanism to protect them from predators and infection. Plants don't have the traditional fight-or-flight options but they do have antinutrients, which either prevent the nutrients in the plant from being absorbed in the gut or act as toxins against predators. The antinutrients, or alkaloids, in the nightshade family are mainly concentrated in the leaves, flowers and unripe fruits, and they're there to make potential predators feel unwell, encouraging them to avoid eating the plant in the future.

For most healthy people nightshades don't pose a problem because a healthy digestive tract prevents absorption of most of the alkaloids. But excessive consumption – if you're eating them every day – can cause a build-up of alkaloids that can take some time to be cleared and may have a negative effect on the body, especially during times of stress.

For those with already-compromised guts and immune systems, and those with an existing autoimmune disease, eating nightshades may create discomfort. A diet high in sugar and refined carbs, especially gluten, seems to exacerbate the problem, as this is thought to alter the gut to the point that it is unable to protect itself from these toxins. When included in a diet high in gluten, sugar and omega 6, potatoes may also have a significant inflammatory effect.

Moral of the story: no matter the phase you're in, if you're suffering from any of the symptoms above or find you aren't making progress, try cutting out the nightshades.

Tips for eating nightshades (if you suspect you are sensitive):

- Don't eat green tomatoes or green or sprouting potatoes;
- Peel your potatoes;
- Only eat very ripe aubergine, and soak the slices in salty water or layer them with salt for a couple of hours before cooking;
- Avoid all processed nightshades, especially those that are deep-fried in seed oils.

ALCOHOL

Alcohol is something of a problem topic.

On the one hand, we're trying to promote health and overall wellbeing, so the advice should be simple: alcohol is a toxin and it's best entirely avoided. On the other hand, booze is also an important social component in many people's lives and ignoring the matter may not be practical or helpful. So what responsible advice can we offer?

The good, the bad and the ugly

On the potential plus side, moderate alcohol consumption – one drink a day for the average woman, two for the average man – may have some health benefits, so if you get it right you can take the edge off *and* hopefully benefit health-wise. That said, the science isn't conclusive; those benefits may be partially or even wholly associated with the type of person who's got their act together to such a degree they can have one drink and then say no more.

In contrast, heavy drinking brings with it a range of potential health problems, from sleep disruption and hangovers to liver disease and certain cancers. It impairs decision-making, encourages risky behaviour and, of course, packs on the weight, with all the associated problems. The guilt of a booze-broken diet is often enough to bring things crashing down to nothing.

We categorically discourage heavy drinking for all these reasons.

What to do?

First of all, realise that drinking alcohol without compromising your health requires discipline. Alcohol is a toxin and alcoholic drinks are usually high in carbohydrates *plus* alcohol gets you drunk – and drunk people make bad decisions. When you're in a sensitive stage of your life – as when undertaking a major lifestyle overhaul! – it's best to make smart decisions with a clear head.

So if you must drink, what should it be?

Avoid normal beer, alcopops, cocktails and spirit mixers – all of which will stop any weight loss dead in its tracks. (Beer is a minefield: you can drink a day's allowance of carbs in one pint and it's often far too tempting to have "just one more". How many slim beer drinkers do you know?)

From a carb-intake perspective we recommend you stick to dry wines (lower sugar content), low-energy (lite) beers and clearer spirits such as gin and vodka. The problem with lite beers is they don't taste great so what's the point? And the problem with spirits is they're often only palatable with a sugar-riddled mixer. So, depending on your preferences, we recommend a glass of half-decent wine with dinner or a whisky – delicious with water, soda, ice or neat – as needed. For many, they are the best practical options. Just remember that you're still consuming (toxic) alcohol.

(Note that when cooking with wine, the alcohol boils away but the carbs remain.)

From a socialising perspective, be mentally prepared when you go to dinners and parties where the drink is likely to flow. When you wing it, you tend to have that glass or three extra you hoped not to. If you have a plan and a ready excuse – "I'm driving" is a good one – it's much easier to make it through in good nick.

The moral of the story: If you can, bin the booze entirely during Restoration and Transformation. Beyond that, if you want to keep alcohol in your life, make a conscious decision to minimise the toxins, minimise the carb intake, and never allow it to be an excuse to make bad diet and lifestyle decisions. In short, drink in moderation. And if you're struggling to lose weight or break through a plateau, forgo alcohol entirely and monitor the effects.

3.2 FAQs

How much fat can I eat?

Remember, the RMR diet (or any LCHF diet) should not be an excuse to gorge on fat. Our fat consumption guidelines vary by phase and individual; see *A note on fats* on p85.

Lots of fat gives me indigestion. What can I do?

As above, the first thing to remember is you don't need to be overdoing the fat. Allow your body to adjust slowly to this new way of eating. But if it's not simply a case of eating too much fat unnecessarily, try the following tips.

If you haven't cooked with much fat in the past, start with coconut oil, which is easily digested by the body.

Try lemon juice or apple cider vinegar in warm water in the mornings and before meals to aid digestion.

Avoid creamy sauces and rather focus on getting your fats from other sources such as avocados, nuts, olive oil, olives, etc.

Gradually add in butter and cheese to see how your body responds.

Which fats can I cook with and which must I avoid?

The best fats to use are coconut oil, olive oil, avocado oil, butter and ghee. Macadamia nut oil also has many health benefits.

Remember, there's no need to go overboard with fats, even the healthy ones.

The fats to avoid at all times are processed vegetable oils such as sunflower and canola oil and margarine.

How much protein can I eat?

Too much protein in your diet isn't recommended; among other things, it can prevent weight loss. As a rule, avoid exceeding more than 30 percent of your daily food intake as protein.

If you're battling to lose weight or haven't got to grips with the ratios of meat to veg, you could follow the guidelines below. One of the complications, though, is working out how much protein there is in each type of food, and it can be difficult to tally it all up. (Steak, for instance, usually contains 25g of protein per 100g. So a 250g steak contains around 60-65g of protein.) As a result, we're not suggesting you count your protein grammage on a daily basis. But when you're starting out you may want to work out roughly how much you should be having during the different phases and try to stay in that region. No need to weigh your food.

Restoration: 1-1.5g of protein per 2lb of Awesome weight.

Transformation: 0.75-1g of protein per 2lb of Awesome weight.

Preservation: 1-1.5g of protein per 2lb of Awesome weight.

If you are trying to build muscle or if you are very active: 1.5-2.2g of protein per 2lb of Awesome weight.

Why's there so much confusion about dairy?

See the entry on dairy on p149.

What about alcohol?

See the entry on alcohol on p152.

How many cappuccinos can I drink in a day?

One cappuccino contains about 7g of carbs, almost all of it in the added milk, so you need to be careful and bear this in mind no matter what phase you're in.

If you are severely insulin resistant and have a lot of weight to lose, we recommend avoiding dairy in your hot drinks until you are close to your ideal body weight. Which means: no cappuccinos during Transformation. If you do have the occasional one be sure to add it to your meal tracker and include it in your total carb count for the day.

A cappuccino a day during Restoration and Preservation should be fine.

Can I follow the RMR diet on a budget?

Yes, you can.

The misconception that LCHF eating can only be achieved at great expense is probably down to two reasons: 1) it *can* be expensive if you're not careful (as most food shopping can be these days), and 2) in comparison, high-carb convenience food is almost always very cheap*.

The first mistake most newbie RMR dieters make is to think they need to stock up on expensive nut flours, coconut oil, nut butters, baked goods, xylitol, etc. You don't need all the fancy stuff to follow this regime properly. Eat lots of vegetables in season; small amounts of protein, including eggs, less expensive cuts of meat (no need for lean fillet and skinless chicken breasts), offal (liver is highly recommended) and less expensive oily fish such as pilchards and sardines (rather than salmon and trout); and render your own fat for cooking. These foods are typically in the order of 10 to 100 times denser in nutritive value than grains – they're just not always conveniently prepared.

In the meantime, realise that carb replacements or alternatives – such as commercial low-carb breads, crackers and pasta – can be expensive but are entirely unnecessary. They're also usually higher in carbs than Green-list foods.

And remember: when you follow this diet right you eat less – which costs less.

---

*The availability of cheap, high-carb convenience food is so pervasive that it helps explain why obesity and its related illnesses are increasingly described as "diseases of poverty". Where once poverty was equated with famine and malnourishment, rising rates of obesity, diabetes, hypertension and hypercholesterolemia are now the mark of emerging economies and the poorer suburbs of First World cities. The ready availability of cheap food laden with sugar and refined carbs is a likely explanation.

What do I do if I can't find or afford the "right" products?

Don't worry about it.

There are various low-carb or "Banting-friendly" products available now, both in supermarkets and speciality stores, and they often come with a premium price tag. Some of them are amazing and some aren't particularly good at all. Remember: the *real* products you need for this diet are the raw ingredients on the Green and Orange lists, most of which are widely available and affordable.

When you do buy "LCHF-friendly" products, don't be fooled by a healthy-sounding name: always check the ingredients.

How can I burn off my belly fat?

The roll of fat around a person's tummy is the most obvious physcial indicator that they suffer from insulin resistance. We call it the insulin roll.

The good news is the RMR diet is perfect for people with an insulin roll. Your best bet is to follow our dietary advice and get stuck into some high-intensity exercise a few times a week. Endurance exercise is less likely to help you lose belly fat.

I have a chronic health condition (epilepsy / type-1 diabetes / type-2 diabetes / cystic fibrosis / high blood pressure / high cholesterol / infertility / dermatitis / etc) and I've heard the RMR diet can help. Is it safe and what must I do to get started?

We believe the answer is yes; the RMR diet may help with all these conditions and more. If you suffer from any medical conditions, though, it is always a good idea to consult a medical practitioner before embarking on a major change to your lifestyle. If you get the go-ahead, go ahead.

Can I continue to train/run/dance/workout when following a strict RMR diet?

In the initial stages of the RMR diet, you may find that you have less energy than usual. To avoid putting unnecessary strain on your body it's best to focus on adjusting to this new way of eating before you include strenuous exercise. Before long you will find you have more energy than ever, and you will want to exercise.

Increasingly, we are hearing from elite and endurance athletes that they are able to perform at their best, even on a strict RMR diet. Some older athletes report recording their best times in a decade or more.

High-profile elite athletes who have reached peak performance on diets with LCHF and Real Meal elements include the likes of sprint icon Usain Bolt (high vegetables and protein); tennis champion Novak Djokovic (gluten-free, low-carb); three-times Tour de France winner Chris Froome; David Pocock, one of the world's best rugby players; and any number of triathletes and endurance runners.

So, go for it!

Is it okay if I miss meals because I'm not hungry?

Absolutely. We recommend only eating when you're hungry. As you adapt to the RMR way of life, you should find yourself naturally eating less anyway. Missing meals is, in fact, a recognised method for countering insulin resistance and encouraging or maintaining weight loss; see *Intermittent Fasting* on p132.

On the other hand, starving yourself – i.e. withholding food to the point where you feel light-headed – is definitely not recommended as that entirely defeats the purpose of being awesome!

Why am I not losing as much weight as others?

Everyone is different and individual responses to the RMR diet (or any way of eating) vary. Don't compare yourself to others; compare yourself to your state of health when you started out, and ensure you're getting healthier and making progress.

An ideal amount to lose is 1-2lb a week. If you're in that range you're doing well. If you get stuck, see *Breaking Through The Plateau* on p139 and *The Awesome Checklist* that follows.

I was losing weight but have now stopped. What's going on?

At the beginning, you may find that you lose weight quickly, but this is likely to be water weight. Expect your weight loss to slow the closer you get to your goal weight; this is normal. If it's stopped for an extended period then you've hit a plateau, for which there could be various reasons. See *Breaking Through The Plateau* on p139 and *The Awesome Checklist* that follows.

Why do men lose weight faster than women?

When it comes to weight loss, it really is a man's world. Unfortunately for women, men tend to lose weight faster because they generally have more muscle, are more emotionally constrained, are genetically wired to handle stress differently and are less likely to have been on as many diets as women. These are all important considerations.

While men generally release stress because of their higher levels of aggression and promiscuity, women tend to be coded to handle stress by putting on weight (which may confer a survival advantage when raising young children). Higher resistance to insulin, often a consequence of yo-yo dieting, also presents a greater challenge when starting the Real Meal Revolution.

In addition to their more complex mix of hormones, women also tend to be more affected by warped social standards that put them under more stress to try to be slim and achieve the ultimate "look". Women who are battling with their weight can suffer from depression, resignation and self-sabotage. It's a minefield.

As above: don't compare yourself to others – it doesn't matter that your partner may be losing weight faster than you; rather compare yourself to your state of health when you started out, and ensure you're getting healthier and making progress. Always emphasise the health aspect over the look – that's just a bonus.

Can I eat this way if I'm pregnant?

We recommend the Restoration or Preservation phases for pregnant or breastfeeding RMR dieters. It is, however, perfectly safe for pregnant mothers to be in ketosis/Transformation; this is vital for type-2 diabetes sufferers, who we believe should remain permanently in this phase.

See *Real Meal Revolution: Raising Superheroes* (Real Meal Revolution, 2015) for more information and recipes for pregnant and breastfeeding mothers. If you have any concerns or questions, see a doctor.

I've fallen off the wagon. How can I get back on?

You're off to a good start simply because you want to get back on it – great going.

If you've had a major crash, start at the beginning with a week of Observation, do a week or two of Restoration and then get stuck into Transformation. If you're attuned to intermittent fasting by this stage, you could start fasting from the get-go. We also highly recommend you join a support group to prevent it from happening again.

If you've had a minor fall – a bad weekend, say – you could skip straight to Transformation and fasting, as recommended on p132.

I often struggle when dining out. What should I order in a restaurant?

Keep your meals simple when eating out. Go for unprocessed proteins and veg like steak or fish with butter and broccoli. A hamburger is an option; just lose the bun and chips. Grilled calamari is good. A major priority is to consciously avoid the extras: sauces, soft drinks, alcohol, dessert.

Here are some more tips:

- Main meal salads are a good option; e.g. chicken Caesar salad.
- Ask for additional salad with other meals.
- Swap potatoes/fries/rice/noodles for vegetables or a salad.
- Ask the waiter to take away the bread basket.
- Avoid breading; e.g. schnitzels and crumbed escalopes.
- Sushi: opt for sashimi or a Japanese salad with salmon or tuna.
- Indian: be wary of the potatoes in curries, not to mention the rice. Avoid poppadums and naan bread.
- Thai: a coconut milk broth with chicken or prawns or a Tom Yum soup is a good choice. Stay away from spring rolls, dim sum, rice and noodle dishes.
- As always, avoid all soft drinks. Rather order sparkling water.

- Be aware of your alcohol intake. Make a conscious decision about how much, if anything, you're going to drink beforehand. If necessary, ask the waiter not to refill your glass. (If you need an excuse, be the designated driver.)

How is a ketogenic diet related to the RMR diet?

When you enter the Transformation phase of Real Meal 2.0, you are effectively following a ketogenic diet. Your body should enter ketosis, which means you are burning fat instead of carbohydrates for fuel. Burning carbs releases glucose into the bloodstream, whereas burning fat releases glucose, fatty acids and ketone bodies into the bloodstream, courtesy of your liver. Most of the organs in the body can use fatty acids for energy, but some, including the brain, can only use either glucose or ketones.

There are two important points to note when your body is in ketosis, i.e. you are following an LCHF diet and transforming your body to preferentially use fat for energy. First, your brain receives plenty of energy from the glucose and ketones being supplied by your liver. In fact, scientists now think the low ratio of glucose in this fuel mix may actually be good for the brain and help protect against disorders such as Alzheimer's and depression.

Second, ketosis is not ketoacidosis. The latter is a rare condition that can occur in patients with type-1 diabetes, or in cases of extreme starvation. For the rest of us, natural mechanisms in our bodies prevent the excessive build-up of ketone bodies in the blood. Being in a state of ketosis is safe and natural.

What about my cholesterol?

The matter of cholesterol is one of the most divisive topics in the modern dietary debate. The entrenched belief, based on the diet-heart hypothesis, claims cholesterol to be bad, end of story: the higher it is, the more likely you are to drop dead from a heart attack. For encouraging a diet that may raise cholesterol levels while frequently querying the effectiveness of statins and other chronic medications, many in the LCHF community have faced savage criticism for supposedly risking people's health. Ironies aside – people are already risking their health when they are obese – the fact of the matter is a) it's more complicated than that, and b) the original entrenched belief has been proven to be wrong.

In the words of Prof Noakes, whose 2012 UCT Faculty of Health Sciences centenary debate was published in the *South African Journal of Clinical Nutrition* in 2015, "Cholesterol is not an important risk factor for heart disease, and the current dietary recommendations do more harm than good."

It is important to realise that cholesterol is imperative for a healthy, functioning body. Ideally, you're aiming for high levels of large, fluffy high-density lipoproteins (HDL), the "good cholesterol", and low levels of small, dense low-density lipoproteins (LDL), "the bad cholesterol". For many people who are following the RMR diet, HDL tends to rise and triglycerides drop, with total and LDL cholesterol tending to stay the same. LDL particle size tends to increase, and LDL particle number tends to go down. These are all good things.

Prof Noakes advises that if you are worried about your cholesterol you should have your triglyceride levels measured; if they are below 1 mmol/L then you can possibly ignore your cholesterol value entirely. If your levels of small dense LDL cholesterol particles are high that is cause for concern. If your total cholesterol is in large, fluffy particles that is good.

Weight loss can result in an increase in cholesterol, a normal response due to the release of fatty acids and triglycerides into the bloodstream, and it is therefore advised to only test your cholesterol once your weight has been stable for at least a month. Either way, high cholesterol is a poor predictor of heart disease; inflammation resulting from a diet high in sugar is now considered the greatest cause of heart disease.

Following the RMR diet reduces inflammation, which improves cholesterol markers in most people, but a small percentage of people do find that their bad cholesterol increases. If you are one of the few who this happens to, we recommend you focus on fats from monounsaturated sources instead of saturated sources.

(For more, read "What to do if your cholesterol increases while Banting" at RealMealRevolution.com.)

There is mounting evidence, now supported by mainstream scientists, that subduing cholesterol levels by taking statins has no significant effect on how much longer men will live, and in the case of women statin therapy may actually be harmful.

In October 2016 Zoe Harcombe went so far as to describe the introduction and prescription of statins as "harmful, and one of the greatest crimes against humanity that the pharmaceutical industry has unleashed".

3.3 OTHER RESOURCES

3.3.1 YOUR INSULIN RESISTANCE AND GENERAL HEALTH

As we noted on p25 in *Who should make the switch?*, we believe that most people will benefit from Real Meal 2.0 to some degree. But the more insulin resistant you are, the more likely you are to benefit (and the more strictly you will have to follow the rules for the best results) from the limited carbohydrates of LCHF eating.

But how do you know how insulin resistant you are?

You can usually get a reasonable sense of your insulin resistance simply by reviewing your weight and personal and family history. See p171 to work out what an ideal weight and hip-waist measurement is for your frame and age, then consider a few things: are you diabetic or pre-diabetic, does diabetes run in your family, do you have a noticeable layer of belly fat and/ or have you steadily put on a couple of pounds or so every year since you were 20? Answer yes to any of those questions, and you're heading towards the "very" category.

But if you're, say, in your thirties and would just like to lose a stone and feel better, it may be difficult to tell. Perhaps you're slightly insulin resistant; perhaps it's the rest of the Pie of Life getting you.

How do you tell?

Well, you can try the RMR diet at a chosen level and observe the effect. Or you could get some blood work done. A common test that many people have at some point is for blood-sugar levels; that is, the amount of glucose in your bloodstream. A normal reading is, of course, better than an elevated reading, but it may not paint the whole picture. If your pancreas is working over time to keep your blood-sugar levels that way, you may still be insulin resistant.

TEST YOUR BLOOD-INSULIN LEVELS

We highly recommend testing your fasting blood-insulin levels. It's a simple blood test that can be performed through your GP or is available privately for around £100. The results should be available within a day.

OTHER BIOMARKER TESTS

Besides measuring your weight, waist-hip ratio, blood pressure, blood-glucose and blood-insulin levels, there are a number of other tests to consider, especially if you have health concerns. To find out more about blood glycated haemoglobin percentage, blood triglyceride concentration, blood HDL-cholesterol concentration and other tests, see RealMealRevolution.com. If you are concerned enough to consider these tests, we do, however, advise you to consult a doctor to learn more.

3.3.2 YOUR PIE CHARTS OF LIFE

For a fuller introduction to the concepts of lifestyle pie charts, refer to *Measuring Your Pie* on p70.

Once you have completed the charts, total up every day in the bottom row, and total up the item on the far right. Each table should give you a clear picture of the things that take up the most of your time, and the people you spend your time with. (We call them pie charts both because they chart the Pie of Life and because you can convert them into actual pie charts at RealMealRevolution.com.)

Make more detailed tables of your own if you'd like to explore this further.

RECORD YOUR PEOPLE PIE TABLE

In the table below, fill in the number of hours you spend with your friends, family, work colleagues and alone. Time in a crowd or on public transport would be considered time spent alone.

	Mon	Tue	Wed	Thu	Fri	Sat	Sun	Total per week
Friends								
Family								
Clients/ Colleagues								
Alone								
TOTAL								

RECORD YOUR ACTIVITY PIE TABLE

In the table below fill in the number of hours you spend participating in the activities listed.

	Mon	Tue	Wed	Thu	Fri	Sat	Sun	Total per week
Work								
Eating & cooking								
Sleeping								
Hobbies								
House work								
Exercise								
Driving								
Watching TV								
Personal development								
Other								
TOTAL								

3.3.3 YOUR AWESOME CHARTS

For a fuller introduction to the concepts of Awesome weight and hip-waist ratios refer to *Getting To Awesome!* on p99.

The charts on the following pages are intended to offer measurement goals for those following an RMR programme that are more accurate than a standard Body Mass Index (BMI) measurement, which makes no allowance for gender or variations in body type. They are, however, still not foolproof. For an even more accurate assessment of your ideal measurements consult a medical expert. And to get an overall Score of Awesomeness, see RealMealRevolution.com.

CALCULATING BODY TYPE

To work out if you are light-, medium- or heavy-framed, wrap your thumb and index finger around the narrowest part of your wrist.

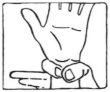

Light frame
finger and thumb
overlap

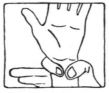

Medium frame
finger and thumb
just touch

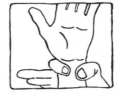

Heavy frame
finger and thumb do
not touch

CALCULATING YOUR AWESOME WEIGHT

To find your target weight (in kg), see the legend over the page, then refer to the tables, cross-referencing your gender, height and body type, and whether or not you have been more than 30 percent overweight in the past.

Ideal weight: an "ideal" or optimum weight that you could reach and maintain if you were saintly with your diet and lifestyle; not actually an ideal weight for most people.
Awesome weight: a healthy weight that you could maintain without letting your diet or lifestyle routines monopolise your time to the detriment of other areas of your life; RMR's recommended weight for most people.

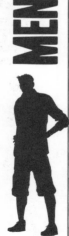

Height	Light framed				Medium framed				Heavy framed			
	Ideal		Awesome		Ideal		Awesome		Ideal		Awesome	
in cm	basic	adjusted	basic	adjusted	basic	adjusted	basic	adjusted	basic	adjusted	basic	adjusted
155	49	50	50	52	52	53	53	55	55	57	57	59
156	50	51	51	53	53	55	55	56	56	58	58	60
157	51	52	52	54	54	56	56	57	57	59	59	61
158	52	53	53	55	55	57	57	58	58	60	60	62
159	53	54	54	56	56	58	58	59	59	61	61	63
160	53	55	55	57	57	59	59	60	60	62	62	64
161	54	56	56	58	58	60	60	61	61	63	63	65
162	55	57	57	59	59	60	60	62	62	64	64	66
163	56	58	58	59	60	61	61	63	63	65	65	67
164	57	59	59	60	61	62	62	64	64	66	66	68
165	58	59	59	61	61	63	63	65	65	67	67	69
166	59	60	60	62	62	64	64	66	66	68	68	70
167	59	61	61	63	63	65	65	67	67	69	69	71
168	60	62	62	64	64	66	66	68	68	70	70	72
169	61	63	63	65	65	67	67	69	69	71	71	73
170	62	64	64	66	66	68	68	70	70	72	72	74
171	63	65	65	67	67	69	69	71	71	73	73	75
172	64	66	66	68	68	70	70	72	72	74	74	76
173	65	66	66	68	69	71	71	73	73	75	75	77
174	65	67	67	69	70	72	72	74	74	76	76	78
175	66	68	68	70	70	73	73	75	75	77	77	79
176	67	69	69	71	71	74	74	76	76	78	78	80
177	68	70	70	72	72	74	74	77	77	79	79	81
178	69	71	71	73	73	75	75	78	78	80	80	82
179	70	72	72	74	74	76	76	79	79	81	81	83
180	70	73	73	75	75	77	77	80	80	82	82	84
181	71	73	73	76	76	78	78	81	80	83	83	85
182	72	74	74	77	77	79	79	81	81	84	84	86
183	73	75	75	77	78	80	80	82	82	85	85	87
184	74	76	76	78	79	81	81	83	83	86	86	88
185	75	77	77	79	80	82	82	84	84	87	87	89
186	76	78	78	80	80	83	83	85	85	88	88	90
187	76	79	79	81	81	84	84	86	86	89	89	91
188	77	80	80	82	82	85	85	87	87	90	90	92
189	78	80	80	83	83	86	86	88	88	91	91	93
190	79	81	81	84	84	87	87	89	89	92	92	95
191	80	82	82	85	85	88	88	90	90	93	93	96
192	81	83	83	86	86	88	88	91	91	94	94	97
193	82	84	84	87	87	89	89	92	92	95	95	98
194	82	85	85	87	88	90	90	93	93	96	96	99
195	83	86	86	88	89	91	91	94	94	97	97	100
196	84	87	87	89	89	92	92	95	95	98	98	101
197	85	88	88	90	90	93	93	96	96	99	99	102
198	86	88	88	91	91	94	94	97	97	100	100	103
199	87	89	89	92	92	95	95	98	98	101	101	104
200	88	90	90	93	93	96	96	99	99	102	102	105

MEN

REAL MEAL 2.0

Basic: your column if you have never been obese.
Adjusted: your column if you have weighed more than 30% more than your Basic weight. For women this excludes weight during pregnancy and three months post-birth.

Height	Light framed				Medium framed				Heavy framed			
	Ideal		Awesome		Ideal		Awesome		Ideal		Awesome	
in cm	basic	adjusted	basic	adjusted	basic	adjusted	basic	adjusted	basic	adjusted	basic	adjusted
155	47	51	48	52	51	55	52	57	55	60	56	62
156	47	52	49	53	51	56	53	58	55	61	57	62
157	48	52	49	54	52	57	54	58	56	61	58	63
158	49	53	50	54	53	57	54	59	57	62	59	64
159	49	54	51	55	53	58	55	60	58	63	59	65
160	50	54	51	56	54	59	56	61	58	64	60	66
161	50	55	54	57	55	60	56	61	59	64	61	66
162	51	56	53	57	55	60	57	62	60	65	62	67
163	52	56	53	58	56	61	58	63	61	66	62	68
164	52	57	54	59	57	62	58	64	61	67	63	69
165	53	58	54	59	57	63	60	64	62	68	64	70
166	53	58	55	60	58	63	60	65	63	68.	65	70
167	54	59	56	61	59	64	61	66	63	69	65	71
168	55	60	56	61	59	65	61	67	64	70	66	72
169	55	60	57	62	60	66	62	67	65	71	67	73
170	56	61	58	63	61	66	63	68	66	72	68	74
171	57	62	58	63	61	67	63	69	66	72	68	75
172	57	62	59	64	62	68	64	70	67	73	69	75
173	58	63	59	65	63	68	65	70	68	74	70	76
174	58	64	60	66	63	69	65	71	69	75	71	77
175	59	64	61	66	64	70	66	72	69	75	71	78
176	60	65	61	67	65	71	67	73	70	76	72	79
177	60	66	62	68	65	71	67	73	71	77	73	79
178	61	66	63	68	66	72	68	74	71	78	74	80
179	61	67	63	69	67	73	69	75	72	79	74	81
180	62	68	64	70	67	74	69	76	73	79	75	82
181	63	68	65	70	68	74	70	77	74	80	76	83
182	63	69	65	71	69	75	71	77	74	81	77	83.
183	64	70	66	72	69	76	72	78	75	82	77	84
184	65	70	66	72	70	76	72	79	76	83	78	85
185	65	71	67	73	71	77	73	80	76	80	79	86
186	66	72	68	74	71	78	74	80	77	84	80	87
187	66	72	68	75	72	79	74	81	78	85	80	87
188	67	73	69	75	73	79	75	82	79	86	81	88
189	68	74	70	76	73	80	76	83	79	87	82	89
190	68	74	70	77	74	81	76	83	80	87	83	90
191	69	75	71	77	75	82	77	84	81	88	83	91
192	69	76	72	78	76	82	78	85	82	89	84	92
193	70	76	72	79	76	83	78	86	82	90	85	92
194	71	77	73	79	77	84	79	86	83	90	85	93
195	71	78	73	80	78	84	80	87	84	91	86	94
196	72	78	74	81	78	85	81	88	84	92	87	95
197	73	79	75	81	79	86	81	89	85	93	88	96
198	73	80	75	82	80	87	82	89	86	94	88.	96
199	74	80	76	83	80	87	83	90	87	94	89	97
200	74	81	77	84	81	88	83	91	87	95	90	98

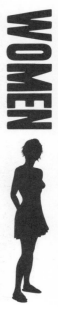

WOMEN

CALCULATING YOUR AWESOME HIP-WAIST RATIO

Divide your waist measurement (taken level across your belly button without letting the tape cut into your flesh) by your hip measurement (taken across the widest part of your hips). Unless you are very overweight the result should be less than 1. Then refer to the tables, cross-referencing your gender and age.

Disease risk related to obesity

	AGE	LOW	MODERATE	HIGH	VERY HIGH
MEN	20-29	< 0.83	0.83-0.88	0.89-0.94	> 0.94
	30-39	< 0.84	0.84-0.91	0.92-0.96	> 0.96
	40-49	< 0.88	0.88-0.95	0.96-1.00	> 1.00
	50-59	< 0.90	0.90-0.96	0.97-1.02	> 1.02
	60-69	< 0.91	0.91-0.98	0.99-1.03	> 1.03
WOMEN	20-29	< 0.71	0.71-0.77	0.78-0.82	> 0.82
	30-39	< 0.72	0.72-0.78	0.79-0.84	> 0.84
	40-49	< 0.73	0.73-0.79	0.80-0.87	> 0.87
	50-59	< 0.74	0.74-0.81	0.82-0.88	> 0.88
	60-69	< 0.76	0.76-0.83	0.84-0.90	> 0.90

3.3.4 THE EXPERTS

As discussed in *A note on the science, resources and referencing* on p27, the information in *The Real Meal Revolution 2.0* (and on our website) owes a great deal to numerous LCHF and nutritional experts around the world. In particular, we follow the doctors, specialists and authors listed over the page, and this list serves as a general resources bibliography for the book. If you're interested in finding out more on a specific health topic, we suggest starting with them.

Of course, our two earlier titles, *The Real Meal Revolution* by Tim Noakes, Jonno Proudfoot, David Grier and Sally-Ann Creed (Quivertree, 2013) and *Real Meal Revolution: Raising Superheroes* by Tim Noakes, Jonno Proudfoot and Bridget Surtees (Real Meal Revolution, 2015), also provided core information. Note that they include numerous Transformation-friendly and Restoration-friendly recipes respectively.

We also gratefully acknowledge the thousands of RMR members who have provided their feedback and thus expanded our knowledge base and contributed to the production of this book.

For a more comprehensive bibliography and more detailed information on the experts, see RealMealRevolution.com.

Ann Childers

🖥 www.lifebalancenw.com 🐦 @AnnChildersMD

Psychiatric physician who specialises in the psychiatric treatment of children, adolescents and adults; member of the American Psychiatric Association, the American Medical Association, the Nutrition and Metabolism Society and the American Society of Bariatric Physicians; expert in the field of nutrition for mental health.

Recommended reading: www.lifebalancenw.com

William Davis

🖥 www.wheatbellyblog.com 🐦 @wheatbelly

Cardiologist and bestselling author who has explored the benefits of cutting wheat from the diet; medical director and founder of the Wheat Belly Lifestyle Institute; seen great success in patients who previously suffered from a variety of chronic illnesses, from arthritis to ulcerative colitis.

Recommended reading: *Wheat Belly* (Rodale, 2011)**;** *Wheat Belly Total Health: The ultimate grain-free health and weight-loss life plan* (Rodale Books, 2014)

Andreas Eenfeldt

🖥 www.dietdoctor.com 🐦 @DietDoctor1

Swedish family doctor who worked in family practice for eight years and treated many obese and pre-diabetic patients using the LCHF diet; currently runs the most successful health blog in Sweden and is the world's most popular LCHF blogger and vlogger.

Recommended reading: *Low Carb, High Fat Food Revolution: Advice and recipes to improve your health and reduce your weight* (Skyhorse Publishing, 2014). Also see www.dietdoctor.com.

Alessio Fasano

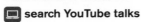 search YouTube talks

World-renowned Italian paediatric gastroenterologist and researcher; currently the chief of paediatric gastroenterology and nutrition at MassGeneral Hospital for Children in Boston, among other positions; expert in leaky gut syndrome, coeliac disease and other gluten-sensitive conditions.

Recommended reading: *Gluten Freedom* (Turner Publishing Co, 2014). Also search his talks online.

Gary Fettke

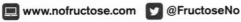 www.nofructose.com @FructoseNo

Orthopaedic surgeon, senior lecturer at the University of Tasmania and Australian campaigner against excess sugar and processed foods; has seen significant improvements in the health of patients prior to surgery as a result of a low-sugar, low-carbohydrate diet; a cancer survivor, he promotes the glucose-cancer model, which hypothesises that fructose and sugar drive cancer.

Recommended reading: www.nofructose.com

Jason Fung
 www.intensivedietarymanagement.com @drjasonfung

Canadian nephrologist, with a particular interest in obesity management; qualifications include nephrology fellowship through the University of California, Los Angeles at the Cedars-Sinai hospital; work and research in kidney care has led to extensive involvement with type-2 diabetes; considered a leading specialist in the use of both LCHF lifestyle and intermittent fasting in the treatment of common diseases.

Recommended reading: *The Obesity Code* (Greystone Books, 2016); *The Complete Guide To Fasting* (with Jimmy Moore; Victory Belt Publishing, 2016). Also search his talks online.

Zoë Harcombe
 www.zoeharcombe.com @zoeharcombe

Long-established researcher in the field of diet and nutrition, who gained her PhD in public health nutrition in 2016; forerunner in LCHF diet research, strong supporter of the inclusion of dietary fat in nutrition and expert at analysing nutrition research. (In October 2016 Harcombe appeared at the HPCSA hearing as an expert witness in defence of Tim Noakes.)

Recommended reading: *Why Do You Overeat? When all you want is to be slim* (Columbus Publishing Ltd, 2012); *The Obesity Epidemic: What caused it? How do we stop it?* (Columbus Publishing Ltd, 2015)

Aseem Malhotra

 www.doctoraseem.com @DrAseemMalhotra

Award-winning cardiologist and expert on treating, diagnosing and preventing heart disease; graduated from the University of Edinburgh and trained at Harefield Hospital in London before working as a doctor in the National Health Service in the United Kingdom; published commentaries have contributed to the prioritisation of sugar reduction in UK dietary guidelines.

Recommended reading: www.draseem.com, his regular blog.

Ted Naiman

www.burnfatnotsugar.com @tednaiman

Medical doctor practising at Virginia Mason Issaquah Medical Center, specialising in family medicine; has used the LCHF diet to treat and cure metabolic diseases such as diabetes and autoimmune diseases; strong supporter of the LCHF lifestyle, advocate for change in nutrition teachings and fan of high-intensity training to assist with weight maintenance.

Recommended reading: www.burnfatnotsugar.com. Also search his talks online.

Tim Noakes

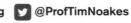 **www.thenoakesfoundation.org** **@ProfTimNoakes**

Emeritus Professor at the University of Cape Town in Exercise Science and Sports Medicine; renowned South African research scientist, chairman of The Noakes Foundation and member of the National Research Foundation of South Africa; the country's leading proponent of the LCHF diet and activist for dietary guideline change.

Recommended reading: *The Real Meal Revolution* (Quivertree, 2013); *The Real Meal Revolution: Raising Superheroes* (The Real Meal Revolution, 2015)

David Perlmutter

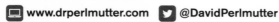 **www.drperlmutter.com** 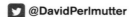 **@DavidPerlmutter**

Medical doctor, board-certified neurologist and Fellow of the American College of Nutrition; recipient of the Linus Pauling Award for his innovative approaches to neurological disorders and the Denham Harman Award for his pioneering work in free radical science and its application in clinical medicine; author of numerous popular books on nutritional influences in neurological disorders.

Recommended reading: *Grain Brain: The surprising truth about wheat, carbs, and sugar – your brain's silent killers* (Yellow Kite Books, 2014)

Stephen Phinney

 www.artandscienceoflowcarb.com

Physician-scientist who has studied and researched at Stanford, MIT and Harvard universities; instrumental in research conducted on diet, exercise, fatty acids and inflammation; all-round LCHF guru. Has worked closely with Jeff Volek and Eric Westman.

Recommended reading: *The New Atkins For A New You: The ultimate diet for shedding weight and feeling great* (Fireside, 2010); *The Art And Science Of Low Carbohydrate Living* (Beyond Obesity LLC, 2011); *The Art And Science Of Low Carbohydrate Performance* (Beyond Obesity LLC, 2012). Also see the documentary *Cereal Killers 2: Run on fat* (2015).

Mark Sisson

 www.marksdailyapple.com @Mark_Sisson

Athlete and endurance marathon runner who has performed independent research on modern diet and nutrition; placed 4th in the 1982 Iron Man World Championship; launched MarksDailyApple.com, a website dedicated to nutrition, exercise and the concept of the Primal Blueprint.

Recommended reading: *The Primal Blueprint* (Primal Nutrition, Inc, 2009)

Gary Taubes

 www.garytaubes.com 🐦 @garytaubes

Award-winning science journalist and author, with master's degrees in aerospace engineering from Stanford and journalism from Columbia; propelled the modern LCHF v LFHC debate into the public domain with his bestselling *Good Calories, Bad Calories*; helped shatter the perceived authority of decades of dietary dogma.

Recommended reading: "What if it's all been a big fat lie?" (2002), available at www.nytimes.com; *Good Calories, Bad Calories: Challenging the conventional wisdom on diet, weight control, and disease* (Alfred A. Knopf, 2007; published as *The Diet Delusion* in the UK); *Why We Get Fat: And what to do about it* (Alfred A Knopf, 2010)

Nina Teicholz

 www.thebigfatsurprise.com 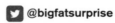 @bigfatsurprise

Investigative journalist; attended Yale and Stanford universities and has a master's from Oxford; bestselling book *The Big Fat Surprise* was named the best science book of 2014 by The Economist and highly praised by *The BMJ, The American Journal of Clinical Nutrition, The Wall Street Journal, Forbes* and others. (In October 2016 Teicholz appeared at the HPCSA hearing as an expert witness in defence of Tim Noakes.)

Recommended reading: *The Big Fat Surprise: Why butter, meat & cheese belong in a healthy diet* (Simon & Schuster, 2014)

Jeff Volek

 www.artandscienceoflowcarb.com

Associate Professor in the Department of Kinesiology at the University of Connecticut; leads a team of researchers specialising in dietary and exercise regimens and nutritional supplements; his studies have shown that the limiting of dietary carbohydrates directly affects weight gain, overall health and athletic performance. Has worked closely with Stephen Phinney and Eric Westman.

Recommended reading: *The New Atkins For A New You: The ultimate diet for shedding weight and feeling great* (Fireside, 2010); *The Art And Science Of Low Carbohydrate Living* (Beyond Obesity LLC, 2011); *The Art And Science Of Low Carbohydrate Performance* (Beyond Obesity LLC, 2012)

Eric Westman

 www.kediet.com

Specialist in the treatment of obesity, diabetes and tobacco dependence; chair of the KE Diet Scientific Advisory Board; associate professor of medicine at Duke University Health System and director of the Duke Lifestyle Medicine Clinic; strong supporter of the ketogenic diet who has received awards and recognition for his contribution to the Obesity Medicine Association. Has worked closely with Stephen Phinney and Jeff Volek.

Recommended reading: *The New Atkins For A New You: The ultimate diet for shedding weight and feeling great* (Fireside, 2010); *A Low Carbohydrate, Ketogenic Diet Manual: No sugar, no starch diet* (CreateSpace Independent Publishing Platform, 2013)

PART 4

RECIPES &

MEAL PLANS

4.1 RMR DIET BASICS

4.2 THE RESTORATION STATION
AND OUR TAKE ON SUPPLEMENTS

4.3 MEAL PLANS

4.1 RMR DIET BASICS

The four recipes below are Real Meal classics; get to know them and making them will become second nature. For a complete list of RMR diet basics, see *The Real Meal Revolution, Raising Superheroes* or RealMealRevolution.com. Note the **Observe** | **Restore** | **Transform** | **Preserve** legend below these basics and the recipes to follow: black means go for it, grey means no.

Seed Crackers (Makes 30 biscuits)

Crackers are good for a quick bite. Play around with the seed proportions.

Ingredients

500ml water
3 tablespoons psyllium husks
200g pumpkin seeds
100g white sesame seeds
70g dark linseeds
10g black sesame seeds
2 teaspoons cumin seeds or fennel seeds (optional)
1 teaspoon salt

Method

- Preheat the oven to 150°C.
- In a bowl, mix the water and psyllium. Leave it to stand for about 10 minutes, at which point it should have thickened to a slimy texture. (Don't panic!)
- In a separate bowl, mix the other ingredients.
- Pour the psyllium water into the seed mixture and combine well.
- Line a baking tray with silicone paper or a silicone mat. (Wax paper doesn't work.)
- Spoon tablespoons of the mixture onto the paper, spreading them into circles about 2mm thick. Make sure there are no holes or bubbles and that you leave about 2cm between the crackers.
- Bake for about 1 hour, or until the crackers are crispy.

OBSERVE | RESTORE | TRANSFORM | PRESERVE

Sesame Biscuits (Makes 50 biscuits)

These biscuits are delicious, but they may need crisping in the oven if they lose their crunch.

Ingredients

300g almond flour/ground almonds
1 ½ teaspoons salt
160g sesame seeds
2 eggs, whisked until frothy
2 tablespoons olive oil

Method

- Preheat the oven to 180°C and grease a baking sheet well or line it with baking paper.
- In a large bowl, mix the almond flour, salt, sesame seeds, eggs and oil. It will form a thick dough, and you may need to get stuck in with your hands to give it a good mix.
- Divide the dough in half.
- Place one half of the dough on a sheet of baking paper and place another sheet over the top. The paper will make it easier to roll out. Using a rolling pin, roll the dough (through the paper) until it's about 2–3mm thick. Remove the top layer of paper and slide the dough onto the baking tray.
- Using a knife or a pizza slicer, slice the dough into 6cm squares.
- Bake for 10–12 minutes, or until golden brown.
- Repeat with the remaining dough.
- Cool and serve. Once cooled, store in an airtight container. If the biscuits soften over time, reheat them in the oven to crisp up.

OBSERVE | RESTORE | TRANSFORM | PRESERVE

Homemade Ketchup (Makes 500ml)

Homemade ketchup is a true winner; the only problem with this recipe is your kids
will want you to make it over and over. It keeps in the fridge for at least two weeks
so make a generous batch.

 Ingredients

50g butter

1 onion, roughly chopped

2 cloves garlic, chopped

½ teaspoon ground ginger

¼ teaspoon ground cinnamon

½ teaspoon ground cloves

¼ teaspoon ground allspice

60g tomato purée

150ml water

200g grated Granny Smith apple, no skin or core

1 x 400g tin whole peeled tomatoes, blended

salt and pepper to taste

1 teaspoon honey (skip during Transformation)

1½ tablespoons apple cider vinegar

 Method

- Heat the butter in a saucepan over a medium heat and gently fry the onion and
  garlic until soft.
- Add the spices and fry for 1 minute, or until they become fragrant.
- Add the tomato purée and cook for another minute until slightly caramelised
  and sweet.
- Add the water, apple and whole peeled tomatoes. Simmer gently over a low
  heat until the mixture has thickened. This will take about an hour.
- Using a hand-blender, blend the sauce until smooth and season well with the
  salt, pepper and honey.
- Add the vinegar and mix thoroughly.
- Place in a clean glass jar, seal and allow it to cool. (Closing the jar while it is still
  hot is the best way to ensure a long shelf life before opening.)
- Keep refrigerated once cooled.

OBSERVE | RESTORE | TRANSFORM | PRESERVE

Homemade Mayo (Makes 375ml)

Homemade mayo isn't just (a lot) better for you than the store-bought stuff, it's better. Period. The key is to not let it terrify you! It's actually quite simple to make once you get the hang of it.

Ingredients

2 egg yolks
3 tablespoons apple cider vinegar (a little less if you want less bite)
1 tablespoon Dijon mustard
½ teaspoon salt
1 clove garlic, grated (optional)
150ml extra virgin olive oil (choose a mild one as the heavy ones can make the mayo bitter)
150ml avocado/macadamia oil, or any other 'fruit' oil with a neutral flavour

Method

- Pour everything except the oils into a bowl.
- Using a hand-blender, mix everything and slowly pour in the oils – the order doesn't matter – in a gentle steady stream, keeping the hand-blender running.
- The mayo will thicken up quite quickly as the oil incorporates; this is what you want. Continue until you've added all the oil.
- If it gets thicker than the mayo you're used to, add a little warm water to thin it out and carry on adding the oils.
- Store in a glass jar in the fridge; it will last for at least two weeks.

Mayo tips

For curry mayo

Add 1 teaspoon curry powder, ½ teaspoon ground turmeric, 1 teaspoon ground coriander, a little honey to taste and a dash of lemon juice. It's also great with some freshly chopped coriander stirred through it.

For tartare sauce

Add some chopped capers, gherkin, spring onion, parsley and a squeeze of lemon.

For lime mayo

Add the zest and juice of 1 juicy lime, and perhaps a bit of chopped chilli.

OBSERVE | RESTORE | TRANSFORM | PRESERVE

4.2 THE RESTORATION STATION
AND OUR TAKE ON REAL SUPPLEMENTS

Every fad diet on the planet is designed to show lightning-fast results in the early days so that dieters think they're on to a winner immediately. They might lose half a stone or so in the first week alone, but then the weight loss typically slows. Real Meal 2.0 disrupts this diet model completely. First, Observation (p104) provides the reality check, then Restoration (p110) primes you for long-term health. Because we're playing the long game, you may lose no weight at all in the first few weeks – don't be alarmed!

LCHF diets that produce dramatic weight loss in the early days tend to pull the classic low-carb move to do so. When you flip into fat-burning mode – as you do on Atkins, South Beach, Dukan and a few other diets, and in Transformation – you stop retaining water, and your initial weight loss is often mostly water loss. (Glucose requires plenty of water to be stored as body fat, and when you initially flush glucose from your system you flush a whole lot of water along with it.) Nothing wrong with the quick weight loss in itself, but as we discussed in Restoration, true sustained weight loss can only occur if your digestive system is in great shape. And when your gut lining has been taking a beating from wheat (gluten), sugar and whatever other nasties you've been consuming, it requires damage control and healing.

By way of analogy, compare your gut to a garden. Imagine you had a vegetable patch with sandy soil that you had been watering with chemical fertiliser for a number of years. You begin to notice that the leaves never look healthy and their colour is a bit off. You also notice the fruit isn't developing properly and the plants aren't growing to their full size.

If you speak to your local nursery and ask for some advice, they might encourage you to start a compost heap and to mix high-quality compost through the bed to improve the general nutrient density and water retention of the soil. In severe cases, the horticulturalist may advise that some of the roots of those plants have been permanently damaged; while you may be able to brighten up the leaves and help the fruit crop improve, the plants may never grow to their full potential.

Your gut is similar. If you're unhealthy and overweight, your gut is likely in distress from having to process all the bad food you've been eating. It needs time, care and fertilisation in order to make the most of the new food that you are putting into it. This can sometimes take up to a year. (In extreme cases, severely compromised people may need to have faecal transplants to repair their bacteria to working order.) Similar to how chemically tainted soil can permanently damage plants' roots to the point that they no longer produce fruit, so your gut lining and bacteria can sustain similar injuries.

Don't fret if you've done a full 12 weeks of Restoration and the pounds aren't falling off as quickly as you'd hoped: you may not have fully repaired your gut for the next phase. It is an ongoing process, and you need to make a habit of taking care of your gut, both as you get into reducing your carb count and in the longer run.

So what do you do?

The more contemporary bio-hackers prescribe a routine of supplements that you often have to take on a daily basis for the rest of your life – both for gut restoration and general health maintenance. We don't disagree that you need these nutrients, but we don't believe it's natural to get the majority of your nutrients from plastic bottles. Wherever possible, we believe it's best to extract all your nutritional needs from real foods. (It's also less expensive.)

BIO-AVAILABILITY IS THE KEY TO NUTRITIONAL INTAKE

Bio-availability refers to how easy it is for your body to actually use the nutrients in something you ingest. For example, if you take an iron supplement you might be taking in 100mg of iron. Due to the nature of the iron, your body may only be able to use 10 percent of that 100mg because that form of iron is not particularly "bio-available". Most real foods, especially lightly cooked vegetables, are far more bio-available.

Below is a list of recommended nutrients as advised by David Perlmutter and others (see *The Experts* from p175). If you are determined to turn around your health and restore your gut, we strongly encourage you to consider getting them into your system.

Easy to get from food, in particular bone broth:
- L-glutamine – improves gut health, among other things. Get it from bone broth, beef, fish, asparagus and cottage cheese.
- Magnesium – boosts energy, improves sleep and reduces muscle cramps and headaches. Get it from foods rich in dietary fibre (prebiotics), such as spinach, broccoli, avocado, nuts and seeds.
- Potassium – reduces fatigue, irritability, muscle cramps and cellulite build-up; most of our organs require it to function. Get it from avocado, spinach, sweet potatoes, kefir, coconut water and mushrooms.
- Collagen – promotes healthy skin and hair, helps with joint lubrication, repairs leaky gut and increases metabolism. Get it from bone broth.
- Glycine – helps cells function correctly and it promotes a healthy digestive, immune and nervous system. Get it from broth, spinach, kale, cauliflower, cabbage, pumpkin, meats, dairy products, eggs, fish and chicken.
- Proline – important for heart health. Get it from bone broth.

Each of these nutrients will have its own guidelines as to what dosage you should take. We're not going to prescribe a dose because we believe you will get more nutrients, and generally more joy, out of getting these nutrients from the real foods in our recipes.

Not as easy to get from food:
- Vitamin D – makes us happy so be sure you're not running low. We used to get it from the sun, but we don't get as much sun as we did (for other health reasons, ironically), and it doesn't exist in a lot of the food we eat.
- B12 – boosts the immune system. People taking the diabetes drug Metformin are at increased risk of developing vitamin B12 deficiency.

If you are deficient in vitamins D and B12 you may require supplements, in which case chat to a healthcare wessional.

REAL SUPPLEMENT RECIPES
The recipes that follow are made to optimise the Restoration phase, and we believe they equal or trump bottled supplements in both nutrient density and deliciousness. You may take a little time getting used to consuming these new foods and drinks on a regular basis, but once your gut bacteria are firing on all cylinders you'll find yourself becoming addicted. Promise.

THE BASICS OF BONE BROTH

Bone broth is a stock, or thin soup, made by simmering bones (beef, chicken or fish) for a lengthy period of time in a liquid flavoured from a base of veggies, herbs and spices. Adding apple cider vinegar helps to extract the minerals and nutrients from the bones while the broth simmers. The slow cooking process preserves the nutrients and, after a decent period of time, allows for collagen to be extracted from the bones, making it gelatinous.

When finished, your broth can be used as the base for soup or gravy or it can be drunk as is – try a little lemon, black pepper and olive oil to season.

Why bone broth?

- The gelatine in bone broth helps protect and heal the mucosal lining of the digestive tract, aiding digestion and neutralising food sensitivities from wheat and dairy. It also helps promote the proliferation of probiotics (good bacteria) in the gut, while reducing inflammation in the digestive tract.
- The glucosamine in bone broth can stimulate the growth of collagen, repair damaged joints and reduce pain and inflammation in the joints.
- The collagen and gelatine in bone broth support hair growth and help strengthen nails.
- The calcium, magnesium, phosphorous and potassium in bone broth help bones grow and repair.
- Bone broth is high in the anti-inflammatory amino acids glycine and proline.
- Glycine can help with sleep and calming the mind.
- Potassium and glycine support cellular and liver detoxification.
- Bone broth supports the immune system and helps fight infections.

How much?

Add a cup of bone broth to your routine every other day, especially in the beginning stages of the RMR diet when your body is relying on the support. Using bone broth to break a fast is also a great hack to save you from eating too much, while ensuring you get heaps of nutrients. It will help your body with hydration and can replenish lost minerals and nutrients, as well as support your gut and immune system. Use the broth as a base for soups, stews, curries and gravies whenever you can. It is a must when you're feeling low and your body is taking a beating from ailments such as a cold or the flu. If you suffer from joint pain we recommend having bone broth daily.

Basic Chicken Broth (Makes about 2 litres)

 Ingredients

1 whole chicken or 1.5kg chicken bones
2.5 litres water
200g carrots, thickly sliced
2 leeks, thinly sliced
1 stalk celery, roughly sliced
2 onions, peeled, studded with 3 cloves
150g button mushrooms, sliced
4 sprigs parsley
2 sprigs thyme
1 bay leaf
5 peppercorns

 Method

- Place the chicken or chicken bones in a large pot and cover with the water.
- Bring to a boil, then turn down to a gentle simmer. Using a slotted spoon, skim off any scum that has risen to the surface.
- Add the remaining ingredients to the stock and simmer gently for 1½–2 hours.
- When it's ready, strain the stock through a fine sieve or muslin cloth. Allow to cool.
- Use immediately or freeze for later use.

OBSERVE | RESTORE | TRANSFORM | PRESERVE

Basic Fish Broth (Makes about 2 litres)

 Ingredients

1kg white fish bones and trimmings
2 tablespoons butter
1 onion, thinly sliced
2 leeks, thinly sliced
4 sprigs parsley
2 sprigs thyme
4 sprigs fennel
1 bay leaf
5 peppercorns
the juice of ½ lemon
2 litres cold water

 Method

- Rinse the fish bones under cold running water and drain.
- Melt the butter in a pot and gently fry the onions and the leeks until completely soft, but not browned.
- Add the remaining ingredients to the pot and bring to a boil.
- Reduce the heat and simmer gently for 25 minutes. Skim off any foam that rises to the top of the liquid.
- When it's ready, strain the stock through a fine sieve or muslin cloth. Allow to cool.
- Use immediately or freeze for later use.

OBSERVE | RESTORE | TRANSFORM | PRESERVE

Basic Beef Broth (Makes about 2 litres)

 Ingredients

1.5kg beef bones
200g carrots, roughly sliced
2 stalks celery, roughly sliced
1 onion, coarsely chopped
2 leeks, thinly sliced
2 litres water (or more)
6 tomatoes, seeded and chopped
150g button mushrooms, thinly sliced
2 cloves garlic, peeled
4 sprigs parsley
2 sprigs thyme
1 bay leaf
5 peppercorns

 Method

- Preheat the oven to 220°C.
- Place the bones in a roasting pan and roast for 30 minutes until well browned, turning occasionally.
- When the bones are brown, add the carrots, celery, onion and leeks to the pan and roast for a further 5 minutes. Give everything a good stir before it goes into the oven.
- Transfer everything from the roasting pan into a large pot, ensuring you scrape out all the flavourful sticky bits.
- Add the remaining ingredients to the pot and cover with water (you could fill the entire pot).
- Bring to a boil. Reduce the heat to a gentle simmer, and simmer uncovered for about 4 hours, skimming off any scum that rises to the surface.
- Strain the stock through a fine sieve or muslin cloth and leave it to cool.
- Use immediately or freeze for later use.

OBSERVE | RESTORE | TRANSFORM | PRESERVE

Chicken Soup for the Soul (makes about 1.5 litres)

Chicken soup for the soul says it all. This is basically a repeat of the original stock-making process, but you are doubling up on the nutrients and flavour.

Ingredients

400g boneless chicken thighs, thinly sliced

1 stick celery, cut into bite-size chunks

3 large leeks, sliced into thick discs

1 massive carrot cut in half, lengthways and then into 1cm-thick pieces

1 litre chicken stock

1 bay leaf

salt and black pepper

1 small handful fresh Italian parsley, roughly chopped

the juice of 1 lemon

Method

- Place everything apart from the seasoning, parsley and lemon into a medium pot.
- Pump the heat up until it hits a rolling boil, then drop it down to a gentle simmer.
- Leave it like that for about an hour, topping up with water if it reduces too much (only top it up to the level at which you started, otherwise you'll dilute it).
- By this point the chicken should be tender and the vegetables should be soft.
- Add the parsley and lemon juice and season with salt and pepper to taste and serve.

Hot tip:

You could add anything else you like to this. Chilli, bacon, cream, mushrooms or anything that takes your fancy.

OBSERVE | RESTORE | TRANSFORM | PRESERVE

Asian Fish Broth (makes about 1.5 litres)

Fish soup is not something everyone feels confident trying. The key is to get the freshest fish humanly possible. With broth especially it doesn't really matter if it's slightly over or undercooked; because it's swimming in soup, it will never dry out. This is a cracker Asian recipe.

 Ingredients

3cm ginger, grated
1 litre fish stock
1 carrot, finely chopped
1 red chilli
6 white radishes, thinly shaved
4 spring onions, finely sliced
2 star anise
6 cloves
400g hake or Cape salmon, cut into 2cm cubes
100g mange tout, sliced julienne
1 handful fresh coriander, roughly chopped
2 tablespoons fish sauce
the juice of 1 lime
sesame seeds

 Method

- Pop the ginger, fish stock, carrot, chilli, radishes, spring onions, star anise and cloves into a medium pot and bang on the heat until the soup begins to simmer.
- Let it simmer for about ten minutes, then add the fish and the mange tout.
- Cook for about 7 to 8 minutes, or until tender.
- Immediately before serving, throw in the coriander, fish sauce, lime juice and sesame seeds.
- If it needs more salt, add more fish sauce. If it needs more sour, add a bit more lime juice.

OBSERVE | RESTORE | TRANSFORM | PRESERVE

Smokey Beef Broth (make about 1.5 litres)

This one's a real fast mover. Make a huge pot of stock on the weekend and you can feed off it three to four times in the week. It saves a heap of time and also saves on cleaning because a broth is typically a one-pot wonder.

 Ingredients

180–250g streaky bacon, chopped into lardons (small pieces)

1 large white onion, finely chopped

1 tablespoon butter

1 large garlic clove, roughly chopped

1 litre beef broth

4 spring onions, finely sliced

10 large cherry tomatoes, cut into quarters

½ teaspoon smoked paprika

1 small handful fresh oregano, picked and roughly chopped

the juice of 1 lemon

salt and pepper

1 red chilli, finely sliced (optional)

 Method

- In a medium-sized pot, over a medium heat, sauté the bacon and onion in the butter until golden brown.
- Once the mixture is golden, toss in the garlic and stir until the mixture becomes fragrant (10–15 minutes).
- By this point, there should be a reasonable sediment formed on the base of the pan. This is where your flavour will come from.
- Pour in the beef broth and increase the heat to full speed until the soup reaches a rolling boil.
- Boil for about 5 minutes and be sure to scrape all the sediment off the bottom of the pan.
- Add the spring onions, cherry tomatoes and smoked paprika and leave to boil for another few minutes.
- You're now pretty much ready to go. Set it aside until just before you eat.
- Before serving, bring back to the boil, add the oregano, lemon juice and season to taste with salt, pepper and chilli (if you're into heat).
- Serve as is.

OBSERVE | RESTORE | TRANSFORM | PRESERVE

APPLE CIDER VINEGAR

Apple cider vinegar is made from fermenting apples. First, the apples or apple cider is exposed to yeast, which ferments the sugars and turns it into alcohol. After a while, a culture of acetic acid and bacteria grows on the surface giving it its sharp, sour taste; this is called the "mother of vinegar".

Apple cider vinegar seems to be more beneficial than other vinegars because it contains acetic acid and the pectin from the apple cider, which is a type of soluble fibre. The more unprocessed and unfiltered your apple cider vinegar is, the better it is for you. If it still contains the "mother", that's even better.

WHY?

- Reduces glucose levels after a meal.
- Reduces the insulin response after a meal.
- Increases satiety, which might make you want to eat less.
- Reduces morning blood-sugar levels in people with type-2 diabetes.
- Lowers triglyceride levels when consumed daily for an extended period of time.

HOW MUCH?

Have two teaspoons just before a meal or with your meal. Or two tablespoons diluted in water before bedtime.

Apple Vinaigrette (makes 500ml)

If you're not into sipping teaspoons of vinegar before meal times, adding it to your diet through dressing is the next best option. Replace your standard French dressing with apple vinaigrette. You don't need to be restricted to salads – dressings like this are great on roasted or steamed veggies too.

 Ingredients

120ml cider vinegar

3 tablespoons Dijon mustard

1 teaspoon honey (skip during Transformation)

1 thumb of ginger grated on a Microplane

240ml avocado oil

120ml extra virgin olive oil

salt and pepper to taste

 Method

- Place the vinegar, mustard, honey and ginger into a mixing bowl and mix well.
- While whisking continuously, pour in the oils until the dressing is emulsified.
- Season with salt and pepper to taste.
- Add a bit more avocado oil if it is too sour. Add some more vinegar if it is too bland (not enough acidity).
- Pour the dressing into a glass bottle with a lid and store in the fridge until needed.

OBSERVE | RESTORE | TRANSFORM | PRESERVE

DIGESTIVE ENZYME-RICH FOODS

Enzymes are necessary for every cell of the body – not just for digestion, but for all physiological processes. Digestive enzyme-rich foods are found naturally in the digestive tract or can be taken in supplement form.

The functions in the body that require enzymes include:
- Energy production
- Oxygen absorption
- Fighting infections and healing wounds
- Reducing inflammation
- Getting nutrients into your cells
- Removing toxic substances
- Breaking down fats, regulating cholesterol and triglyceride levels
- Dissolving blood clots
- Proper hormone regulation
- Slowing the ageing process

Digestive enzymes break down food into amino acids, fatty acids, cholesterol, simple sugars and nucleic acids, which help make DNA.

WHY DIGESTIVE ENZYMES?
- Can take stress off the stomach, pancreas, liver, gall bladder and small intestine by breaking down hard-to-digest proteins, carbohydrates and fats.
- Help heal leaky gut, assist the body in breaking down difficult-to-digest proteins and sugars such as gluten, casein and lactose.
- Improve symptoms of acid reflux and IBS, enhance nutrition absorption and prevent nutritional deficiency.
- If you have a compromised digestive system (leaky gut, IBS, bloating, gas, acid reflux, ulcerative colitis, diarrhoea, constipation, malabsorption), it might be necessary to increase your intake of digestive enzymes.

HOW MUCH?
It depends on how well your bowels are working. If you're having regular bowel movements, you may be okay. However, if you're in need of some digestive assistance, you could add these enzymes if and when needed.

When you switch to low-carb, you are likely to find yourself constipated at least once or twice (and for some it may intially be quite severe). These foods will quickly sort that out for you. Remember that limiting carbohydrates still applies, regardless of the digestive enzymes, so cater for the carbohydrates in the fruits in your daily allowance (count them as your 30g for the day).

- Papaya – try mixing a few tablespoons with kefir and ice in a smoothie.
- Pineapple – you could eat this chargrilled in a salad or in a smoothie as above.
- Avocado – eat as is or in every salad, smoothie or shake you have.
- Extra virgin olive oil and coconut oil – use this in all of your cooking and/ or dressings.
- Raw meat – make sure your source is hygienic, then enjoy sashimi, carpaccio and steak tartare.

FIBRE-RICH (PREBIOTIC) FOODS

Prebiotic foods are foods high in fibre. There are heaps of them available and most of them sit on our Green and Orange lists. Look out for ingredients labelled with 'P'. These are high in fibre and are just what your gut needs to rock and roll.

Here is a list of some of our favourites for ease of reference:
Avocado, asparagus, artichokes, basil, beans, berries, cabbage, carrots, fruit and vegetables with skins, garlic, gem squash, leafy greens like kale, chard, spinach, broccoli and cauliflower, leeks, nuts, onion, oregano, parsley, peppers, radishes, sesame seeds, sunflower seeds, sweet potatoes.

Supplements: You can supplement with fibre like psyllium husks, but this will not provide the nutrients that vegetables will.

WHY PREBIOTIC FOODS?
- Feed the good gut bacteria, which improves not only digestion but overall health.
- Help to reduce carb absorption, lower blood sugar and insulin and therefore help protect against insulin resistance.
- Slow down food absorption, leaving you fuller for longer.
- Stimulate more effective peristalsis, which moves foods through the intestine, ensuring optimal absorption of nutrients while getting rid of any toxins and undigested food.

HOW MUCH?
Aim for at least one cup a day, but three is preferable (depending on your phase and required carb count).

TURMERIC

Turmeric is a yellow spice, usually found in curries, that has been found to have many health benefits due to the active ingredient curcumin. There have been thousands of peer-reviewed articles indicating the benefits of turmeric and curcumin, and various studies report that curcumin is more effective than some prescription drugs at tackling inflammation. This is predominantly because there are fewer side effects when consuming curcumin, unless you are taking it excessively.

WHY TURMERIC?

- Massive anti-inflammatory and anti-cancer properties.
- Aids digestion.
- Helps to reduce blood-sugar levels, thus lowering the risk of diabetes and insulin resistance.
- Associated with the relief of symptoms of depression, arthritis, high cholesterol and chronic pain.

DISCLAIMER: Turmeric may interfere with anti-coagulants like Clopidogrel, Aspirin and Warfarin. It also can affect medications such as non-steroidal, anti-inflammatory drugs. If you are taking any chronic medications or suffer from any chronic medical conditions, speak to your doctor or healthcare provider before introducing large amounts of turmeric into your diet.

HOW MUCH?

Try to add turmeric to your diet at least three times a week. A regular turmeric capsule is also an option; we don't consider this a bottled supplement because it's literally just a capsule of the spice, not a processed extract. Think of it as capsule of basil or parsley.

Golden Shake (Makes one portion, or one dose of turmeric)

As we've said, taking a turmeric supplement is fine, but if you want to have your turmeric in a slightly more exciting fashion, a drink like the one here is a delicious alternative. Have it hot or cold, but only heat it if you're using the coconut milk option; warming the kefir will kill its bacteria.

Ingredients
250ml milk kefir (cold only) or coconut milk (hot or cold)
½ teaspoon turmeric
¼ teaspoon Ceylon cinnamon
1 teaspoon chia seeds
½ teaspoon maca powder
a crack of black pepper
a pinch of crystal salt
½ teaspoon honey (skip during Transformation)

Method
- Warm the milk on the stove (hot option only).
- Combine all the ingredients and blend, in descending ease of use, in a Nutribullet, with a stick blender or in any other blender.

OBSERVE | RESTORE | TRANSFORM | PRESERVE

PROBIOTIC-RICH FOODS & DRINKS

As discussed in *Fermented foods v probiotics* on p116, we encourage the consumption of fermented probiotic-rich foods on a daily basis rather than the ongoing use of probiotic supplements. Fermented foods include natural brine-fermented pickles, sauerkraut and kimchi, and fermented drinks include kefir, kombucha, naturally fermented buttermilk and amasi.

WHY PROBIOTIC-RICH FOODS?

- Replenish and restore balance of the gut biome.
- Reduce food sensitivities.
- Reduce inflammation.
- Reduce intestinal permeability. (A healthy digestive tract reduces toxin absorption and the propensity for auto-immune disease.)
- Increase nutrient absorption.
- Assist in weight loss.
- Help digest and assimilate your food.
- Influence the activity of hundreds of genes.

Basically, a balanced gut biome is the ticket to supreme health. There are not enough pages in this section to explain just how important it is but if you've read the rest of this book you'll have a pretty good idea.

HOW MUCH?

- Probiotic supplements – take whatever your doctor prescribes (if, for instance, you're on antibiotics) or whatever it says on the bottle.

Note: Because of death by stomach acid, the bacteria in supplements often don't make it to the colon, which is where you want them. Fermented foods, in contrast, provide a protective layer to the bacteria and thus help them get where they need to go. Fermented foods are the long-term solution, but taking a supplement for the first 30 days on Real Meal 2.0 will help to kick-start the proliferation of good gut bacteria. Also, if you have a compromised immune system as a result of taking antibiotics, travelling to foreign countries, eating at unknown restaurants, are under great stress, have had recent food poisoning or gastroenteritis, or another illness including flu or a yeast infection such as candida, it is recommended that you take a probiotic supplement in conjunction with probiotic-rich foods and drinks for an added immune boost – even if it's just while you're getting into the swing of things.

When you do require a probiotic supplement, it should be a high-quality, multi-species probiotic. Look for supplements that contain lactobacillus, acidophilus and bifidobacteria in the billions. You will only find high-quality probiotics in the refrigerator and the best are in liquid form.

■ Fermented foods – start off with a teaspoon at every meal for one or two days and monitor your body's reaction. If you encounter bloating and abdominal discomfort, switch to once every three days until the symptoms subside. Then up the dose.

■ Fermented drinks – start off with a quarter of a cup of kefir or half a cup of kombucha per day and monitor your body's reaction. If you encounter light bloating and abdominal discomfort, lower your intake until you find a sweet spot that doesn't stimulate the above.

The maximum, or recommended, amount to end up on would be about one glass of kombucha or kefir per day, along with one portion of fermented veg every couple of days, or vice versa. Just like that healthy soil in your vegetable garden, you need to keep fertilising your gut.

You could skip the drink one day and have more vegetables, or the standard serving of vegetables. It's not clinical medicine, so you can't overdose or underdose. It is more like watering a garden. If you miss a day don't drown the plants the next day; pick it up again, carry on – and just ensure you're not poisoning your plants!

KOMBUCHA

Classic kombucha is a fermented black tea with Eastern origins, and there is something about this naturally fizzy drink that has trendy kids all over the world wildly excited. As a result of fermentation, it is rich in nutrients and healthy bacteria which, for our purposes, makes it perfect for daily consumption during Restoration and Preservation.

Unlike beer or wine, which make use of yeast alone, the fermentation aid in kombucha is a jelly-like mushroom called a scoby, short for "symbiotic colony of bacteria and yeast". If you buy kombucha from any health shop, you can make your own scoby, provided the stuff you're buying is high-enough quality. Or you could get one from a friend who brews it. Either way, making your own scoby and kombucha is preferable when following the RMR diet because it allows you more control over the sugar content – plus it is considerably less expensive.

The fermentation process is the key, converting sugar into nutrients and bacteria, but it isn't an exact science, with timings dependent on different climates, room temperatures and other factors. You can tell your kombucha isn't fermented enough if it's still sweet to the taste. Remember, without sufficient fermentation, you're simply drinking a sugary drink – not what we're looking for! You will know your kombucha is ready to drink when it tastes sour – almost free from any kind of sweetness. If you want to get technical, you could test it for sugar content, but that's unnecessary for even an enthusiastic kombucha fan.

Kombucha is suitable during Restoration and Preservation because during these phases you will have a firm grasp on your carb intake and the effect it has on your body and you won't be too concerned with counting the carbs. Because of the temperamental sugar content, we don't recommend drinking kombucha during Transformation – or ever if you are type-2 diabetic or highly insulin resistant.

Making the scoby

Ingredients

2.5 litres water
6 teabags (Five Roses, Earl Grey or any Asian black tea)
200g white sugar
1 bottle (350–500ml) store-bought live kombucha

Utensils

A 3-litre jar
A 400ml jar (or any small jar)
A muslin cloth

Method

- Make sure the large jar is clean and sterilised.
- Boil the water (either in the kettle or in a pot).
- Place the teabags and sugar into the jar.
- Pour the boiling water over the tea and the sugar, stir gently and leave to brew and cool (essentially making one massive cup of tea).
- Once the tea is cool, remove the teabags.
- Pour in the bottle of kombucha. Remove some of the tea to make space if necessary.
- Cover the opening of the jar with the muslin cloth and fasten it with an elastic band.
- Leave the jar at room temperature for about two weeks.
- A thick layer of jelly-like "scoby" will form either at the bottom or around the opening of the jar. It should be the same texture as thick, overcooked lasagne sheets.
- To harvest the scoby, use a pair of tongs to lift it into the small clean sterile jar and cover it with some leftover "tea" from your main batch. You can leave it in the tea for up to two weeks before using it to make your next batch.
- Note: The tea that is left in your big jar is your first batch of kombucha. You can bottle it, decant it into jugs or just leave it in the jar.

OBSERVE | RESTORE | TRANSFORM | PRESERVE

Making the kombucha (using your own scoby)

Ingredients
3 litres water
6 teabags (for more tannin and caffeine use black tea, Earl Grey or Five Roses. For something different use Rooibos)
200g white sugar
1 scoby (the kombucha mushroom)
250ml kombucha (from a bottle or previous batch)

Utensils
3-litre jar

Method
- Make sure your jar is clean and rinsed of detergent.
- Boil the water.
- Place the teabags, sugar and any flavour combinations (see below) into the jar.
- Pour in the boiling water, stir gently to dissolve the sugar, and leave to brew and cool (making your one massive cup of tea).
- Wait until the mixture is cold.
- Add the scoby and the old kombucha.
- Cover it with a cloth and leave to ferment for a week in winter and three days in summer.

Some flavour combinations
Always add the flavours just before you add the hot water.

- Lemon and bay – add the zest of one big lemon and two fresh bay leaves
- Lavender and lemongrass – 1 stick lemongrass cut in half lengthways and 30cm lavender
- Rosemary and lemon – 20cm rosemary and the zest of one big lemon
- Ginger – 80g fresh ginger sliced lengthways into 2mm matchsticks
- Chai – 4 additional chai teabags
- Cinnamon – 2 sticks cinnamon (not the bark)

The kombucha-making lowdown

During fermentation, the scoby may float to the top or sit at the bottom – don't worry, either way.

Taste the kombucha before bottling. It should be crisp, refreshing and quite tart, with a slight fizz and only a very little sweetness on the palate. Because of the added sugar, it can sometimes be too sweet – in which case let it ferment a bit longer to allow the bacteria to eat more of the sugar as part of the fermentation process. As it gets older, the kombucha will get fizzier and dryer (more sour). If you're worried about your carb count, wait three weeks to get a very crisp, non-sweet kombucha.

Before you bottle it, remove the scoby and store it in a jar with a cup of kombucha covering it to keep it alive.

Start small. Have a shot twice a day. Try get up to a cup or two per day.

Notes on bottling

- Make sure your bottles are clean.
- Decant the batch into another vessel before bottling to get rid of the scum.
- Pour the clear kombucha off the top of your batch through a sieve and a muslin cloth. Stop pouring just before the scum from the bottom gets to the rim of the jar and discard the bit that stays behind.
- Pour the tea into each bottle using a funnel and jug.
- You can bottle in plastic or glass, but be aware the bottles may eventually explode so don't leave them for too long, especially if using glass.
- Make sure you date the bottle so you know which ones are older and more likely to explode and which will most likely have a lower sugar content.

Sauerkraut

Sauerkraut is one of the best known probiotics – if not the best – available. Lab tests on bacteria quantities in this German speciality come back with some astonishing results: in one estimate, a handful of well-matured sauerkraut contained more bacteria than 90 good-quality probiotic capsules. Moreover, the cell walls and rigid casings of sauerkraut are thought to protect the bacteria on their journey through the gut to the colon, which is where they do their work.

Note: bottled or tinned sauerkraut that contains any sugar or vinegar is not sauerkraut. True sauerkraut gets its sweet and sour flavour from natural fermentation. If you are eating store-bought sauerkraut that came pre-packaged and isn't "live", you may achieve the opposite of your intended result.

Ingredients

1 head cabbage
3 heaped teaspoons fine salt

Method

- Shred the cabbage as finely as possible and place it in a large mixing bowl.
- Sprinkle the salt evenly over the cabbage, then use clean hands to crush the cabbage and salt together to draw out the moisture. It should become quite wet and juicy.
- Decant the cabbage into a ceramic sauerkraut crock or "fermenting container" and push the cabbage beneath the surface of the liquid.
- You can press the cabbage under the liquid using a weighted plate. Ensure it's fully submerged (topping it up with a little water if necessary), otherwise it could spoil.
- Leave the cabbage like that for up to ten days, by which point it should be fermented.
- Decant it into a clean container, removing any scummy or mouldy bits.
- You can eat it immediately but it will get better and better with age.

OBSERVE | RESTORE | TRANSFORM | PRESERVE

Mads's Kimchi

I met Madeleine in the very first support group I ran with my friend Rob Hichens. A few months after she left the group, she popped in with a present: the most amazing jar of kimchi. It was so flipping delicious we asked her if she wouldn't mind donating her recipe to the rest of the world. Thanks, Mads. You're a legend!

Ingredients
1 Chinese cabbage, cut into 4cm strips
60g salt (local and natural is always better)
20ml roughly chopped garlic
30ml roughly chopped ginger
50ml sriracha (a hot Thai chilli sauce)
50ml fish sauce
30ml vinegar (I use organic apple cider vinegar to help with the fermentation)
20ml dried chilli flakes
1 teaspoon sugar (up this to 2 teaspoons sugar for an extra-sour kimchi – it ferments, don't worry)
12 radishes, finely sliced
4 spring onions, chopped

Method
- Place the cabbage into a large bowl and cover it with salt, ensuring all the pieces are evenly coated.
- Add just enough water to cover cabbage and weigh it down with a plate or smaller bowl to ensure all the cabbage is immersed in the water.
- Soak for 2 hours.
- Rinse the cabbage under clean running cold water until all the salt is washed away. Squeeze any excess water from the cabbage.
- Mix all the other ingredients except the radishes and spring onions and rub into the cabbage, trying to ensure even distribution.
- Add the radishes and spring onions and mix well.
- Press as tightly as possible into a jar with a tight-fitting lid to compress the ingredients. The tighter the better, as you want as little air in the jar as possible.
- Seal and open every few hours and press further down – the liquid will increase as the cabbage weeps – this is the good stuff so don't throw it out!
- Leave at room temperature for at least seven days, after which you can refrigerate.

OBSERVE | RESTORE | TRANSFORM | PRESERVE

Milk Kefir

Milk kefir, made from cultured kefir grains, is one of the healthiest dairy drinks. This is because the fermentation process reduces the lactose (sugar) content of the milk, a good thing in itself and because it means you're less likely to react if lactose intolerant. The longer you let it ferment, the lower the lactose content, but the more sour it will be too. You can make kefir by simply adding the kefir granules to a glass of milk, or by adding them to other dairy products like sour cream. You can then use the fermented goods in other recipes to add a kick of probiotics and flavour.

An added bonus of milk kefir: if you are totally lactose intolerant you can use coconut milk instead of ordinary milk.

Ingredients
kefir grains
milk

Utensils
1 jar (approx. 1 litre)

Method
- Put the kefir grains into a jar.
- Slowly add the milk while stirring the mixture with a wooden spoon.
- Cover lightly and allow 12–24 hours for culturing, depending on room temperature and the flavour you're after.

How to use
This healthy drink can be enjoyed in so many ways. Drink it as is, munch in a bowl with some fruit and nuts, or blend it and use as a base for a power smoothie.

OBSERVE | RESTORE | TRANSFORM | PRESERVE

Kefired Sour Cream

 Ingredients
kefir grains
cream

 Utensils
1 jar (approx. 1 litre)

Method
- Put the kefir grains into a jar.
- Slowly add the cream while stirring the mixture with a wooden spoon.
- Cover and allow 12–24 hours for culturing, depending on room temperature and desired flavour. It will turn into a gobsmackingly tangy, sour cream.

How to use it

This works well with tacos, soups and desserts – you can smother just about anything with this deliciously cultured dairy product. Even use it as the base for a show-stopper vegetable dip or salad dressing. For a crowd-pleaser – a dip to end all dips – add some fried bacon bits and fat to your kefired sour cream.

Kefir Butter

 Ingredients
kefired sour cream

Method
- Beat kefired sour cream until the butter fat separates from the buttermilk.
- Wash and rinse as you usually would.

How to use it

Your kefir butter will be rich, nutty and cultured, similar in taste to the butter often found in Europe. Cook with it, spread it on gluten-free/LCHF bread or use in your favourite icing recipes. Go wild! And note that it keeps longer than normal butter.

OBSERVE | RESTORE | TRANSFORM | PRESERVE

Soft Kefir Cheese

Ingredients
milk kefir

Method
- Put the milk kefir into a sieve lined with either cheesecloth, a paper coffee filter or a clean tea towel.
- Allow to stand and drain over a bowl for 6–12 hours, or until it has the texture of cream cheese.

How to use it
Enjoy this cultured cheese on gluten-free/LCHF toast or add it to chopped herbs and garlic for a moreish spread or party dip. It also makes a great replacement for mayonnaise in a potato salad.

Hard Kefir Cheese
Hard kefir cheese is simply the next step along from the soft variety.

Ingredients
milk kefir

Method
- Wrap soft kefir cheese in cheesecloth or a tea towel and place it in a colander.
- Weigh down the cheese by covering with a plate under something fairly light, like a can of beans. Continue adding more weight every couple hours until the dripping stops.

How to use it
This crumbly cheese is best enjoyed grated over soups, salads, sandwiches, pizzas, vegetables or anything else that could use a tangy, creamy flavour kick.

OBSERVE | RESTORE | TRANSFORM | PRESERVE

Water Kefir (makes approximately 1 litre)

In general, water kefir is high in sugar even after a long fermentation. In my experience, I have still not tasted a very dry water kefir. For this reason, we can't recommend drinking water kefir during Transformation, but we certainly recommend picking it up during Preservation.

Ingredients

50g sugar
hot water
a pinch of bicarbonate of soda or sea salt (if you have carbon-filtered water)
kefir grains

Utensils

Jar

Method

- Mix the sugar with just enough hot water for it to dissolve.
- Add cool water to fill the jar, leaving 3–4cm at the top.
- Add the sea salt or bicarbonate of soda to the mixture.
- Add the kefir grains once the water has cooled to room temperature.
- Cover the jar tightly with a towel or filter held tightly in place with a rubber band. Allow 24–48 hours for culturing. (24 hours of culturing will yield a sweeter flavour, and after 48 hours the grains will consume a larger portion of the sugar.)
- Once cultured, use a fine mesh plastic or stainless steel strainer when you transfer the liquid into a separate container. Cover with a tight-fitting lid.

How to use it

- Enjoy your water kefir on its own as a nutritious, immune-boosting drink, or add homemade flavouring of your choice. If you wish to drink your water kefir on its own, you'll probably prefer less cultured kefir (24 hours), which is slightly sweeter.
- Finished water kefir does not require refrigeration, but it can be refrigerated if you would rather consume it cold.

OBSERVE | RESTORE | TRANSFORM | **PRESERVE**

FERMENTED PICKLES

The gherkin is the most popular brined pickle on Earth. Before the food corporates got hold of them and started using vinegar and sugar to add fake sweet-and-sourness, all of the tanginess came from natural fermentation in a brine solution. We suggest getting back to the homemade versions.

Before you do, though, a note on brine. The brine recipe over the page has a 7 percent salt content. In colder climates, it is safe to use lower-salt brine, at 4 or 5 percent. In warmer places, the slightly higher salt content controls the fermentation, keeping things from getting too wild in the jar.

Pickle spice mixture

This is a simple spice mixture you can use to pickle just about anything. But the spices are entirely up to you. If you wanted, you could just use a teaspoon of mustard seeds – whatever is convenient or takes your fancy.

 Ingredients

1 stick cinnamon, broken up

1 tablespoon black peppercorns

1 tablespoon yellow mustard seeds

1 teaspoon fennel seeds

2 teaspoons whole allspice

2 teaspoons whole coriander

1 tablespoon dill seeds

 Method

■ Place all the ingredients in a jar and store.

OBSERVE | RESTORE | TRANSFORM | PRESERVE

A basic pickle

You can use this brine on absolutely any vegetable you would like to pickle.

Ingredients

For the brine:
1 litre water
7% salt (natural and local is always better)

For the pickle:
1kg vegetables (we suggest starting with cucumbers or cauliflower)
1 tablespoon pickling spice mixture of your choice (see previous page)
1 vine leaf (not essential)

Method

- In a small saucepan, bring the water, salt and spices to a boil. Leave them to cool.
- Pack the veg as tightly as possible into sterilised jars and cover with brine, making sure there is a piece of vine leaf in each jar.
- Leave the jars at room temperature (18–22°C) for three or four days. Bubbles will begin forming. This is normal; just skim them off and top up with more water or brine if you need to.
- Initially, you may need to weigh the veg down with another jar to keep them submerged. Once the fermentation gets deep into the flesh, they will start sinking.
- After three weeks, your pickles should be ready.
- Keep them in the fridge from this point with the lids on. From here on, they will stay edible while they slowly continue to ferment.
- To keep them fresh longer, you can drain and transfer them to new sterilised jars. Bring the same pickling brine to a boil, pour it back over them in the jars, then seal.
- When they are ready, the vegetables should be opaque, crunchy and tart.
- Slimy, mushy veggies are the result of botched fermentation and are spoilt. Sadly, you'll have to chuck them and start over.

Note: The vine leaves are an insurance policy. They help keep the pickles fresh and crunchy. The fermenting brine is very nutritious and is said to be an epic hangover cure. Some dried or fresh chilli in the pickling mix would also add a nice kick.

OBSERVE | RESTORE | TRANSFORM | PRESERVE

A FINAL NOTE ON MAKING YOUR OWN FOOD

Eating on the RMR diet does not have to be expensive. There are many different ways to follow the RMR rules, according to your income. You could, for instance, live solely on chicken necks and sauerkraut, which is basically what most of South Africa survives on (minus the mealie meal).

Product lines can be fantastic. They provide people with options that may otherwise be difficult for them to get. But just because the product is available doesn't mean we need to excessively consume it. At Real Meal Revolution we don't believe that eating anything in excessive amounts will help you lose weight or get healthy. Actually, eating less, provided what you're eating is outrageously healthy, is by far the best way to improve your health.

If I were a businessman running a food-product business, I would be hell-bent on encouraging people to consume more – but this goes against everything the Real Meal Revolution stands for. This is why we prefer to teach people how to cook. Making your own food puts the power in your hands.

IN SUMMARY

- Consider taking a daily vitamin D and a vitamin B12 supplement; otherwise do your best to consume real-food supplements rather than the bottled kind.
- Eat fibre-rich foods every day.
- Take a turmeric capsule or eat turmeric often.
- Eat a small portion of fermented food every day, or every other day. Then increase according to your palate.
- Drink a small portion of bone broth every other day – ideally alternating between broth and fermented foods.
- Eat foods high in digestive enzymes as often as possible.
- Enjoy preparing, sharing and benefiting from real food and real nutrition!

	BREAKFAST	LUNCH	SUPPER
MONDAY Carbs: 46–52g Fat: 133–152g Protein: 91–110g	2–3 egg omelette/fried eggs in butter with cheese, red pepper, tomato and sautéed onion	½–⅔ tin tuna in brine with 2–3 tbsp mayo, ½–¾ avocado, ¼ mango diced (optional), diced cucumber with salad dressed with olive oil and apple cider vinegar/apple vinaigrette	½–1 cup mince (made with onion, tomato purée/tinned tomatoes, seasoning and green-listed veg) topped with ½–1 cup cauli-mash and minimum 1 cup broccoli
TUESDAY Carbs: 57–58g Fat: 128–143g Protein: 99–118g	¼ cup granola (toast a mixture of nuts and seeds with some spices) with 1 cup yoghurt/kefir, ¼ papaya and 1–2 boiled eggs	Leftover ½–1 cup mince (made with onion, tomato purée/tinned tomatoes, seasoning and green-listed veg) topped with ½–1 cup cauli-mash and minimum 1 cup broccoli	100–120g portion grilled/roast chicken with ½ cup roasted pumpkin, ½ cup green beans, ¼ roasted sweet potato, and gravy made from pan juices (reduce with a dollop of cream and butter)
WEDNESDAY Carbs: 40–42g Fat: 137–157g Protein: 86–104g	2 egg omelette with filling of 1 bacon rasher, Swiss chard, cheese, broccoli and mushrooms with a rocket and tomato salad	Salad with 50–70g leftover chicken, brined pickles, ½ cup asparagus, boiled egg and 2–3 tbsp mayo	100–120g grilled salmon fillet with ½ cup sweet potato, 1 cup green-listed veg with homemade cream lemon-butter sauce (make a lemon butter and then add a dollop of cream to finish), with capers (optional)
THURSDAY Carbs: 58–60g Fat: 129–149g Protein: 113–121g	¼ cup granola (toast a mixture of nuts and seeds with some spices) with 1 cup yoghurt/kefir, ¼ mango and 1–2 boiled eggs	Tuna/egg mayo (½ tin tuna / 2 boiled eggs), 2 tbsp mayo, with ½–1 avocado, radishes, brined pickles, watercress and Seed Crackers	Crispy grilled pork chop with a mixture of sautéed onion, fennel and apple and ½ cup cauli-mash and ¼ cup sauerkraut, with a gravy made from pan juices and chicken stock
FRIDAY Carbs: 62–72g Fat:113–128g Protein: 110–129g	2–3 fried eggs with ½ avocado, grilled tomato and grated cheese	Leftover crispy grilled pork chop with a mixture of sautéed onion, fennel and apple, ½ cup cauli-mash and ¼ cup sauerkraut, with a gravy made from pan juices and chicken stock	Grilled white fish fillet (100–120g) with a few sweet potato wedges, ½ cup peas and ¼ cup sauerkraut/kimchi
SATURDAY Carbs: 46–48g Fat: 158–189g Protein: 114–138g	2–3 eggs scrambled with 1–2 pork/beef sausages (no fillers) with sautéed spinach and grated cheese	2 fish cakes made with leftover fish and mayo on crunchy salad of spinach, red cabbage, grated carrot and radish with an olive oil and apple cider dressing/apple vinaigrette	1–2 Low-carb pancakes filled with spicy mince, with ½ smashed avocado, 1–2 tbsp sour cream/kefired sour cream and grated cheese
SUNDAY Carbs: 63–87g Fat: 117–125g Protein: 91–99g	2–3 low-carb pancakes with 1–1.5 small bananas, 2–3 tbsp nut butter, cinnamon and a dollop of yoghurt with 2 rashers crispy bacon	Leftover spicy mince on ½–1 buttered sweet potato with ½ smashed avocado, 1–2 tbsp sour cream/kefired sour cream and grated cheese	100–120g grilled chicken breast with sautéed mushrooms and peppers on a bed of courgette noodles with a squeeze of lemon and a pat of butter

DRINKS	SNACKS	TIPS	LIFESTYLE TIPS
■ 2 black coffees a day or 4 cups of black tea* ■ Unlimited water or herbal teas *can add cream to coffee and tea	Smoothie made with ¼ cup coconut milk, ¼ cup yoghurt/kefir, ¼ cup blueberries	Make a batch of mayo on Sunday for the week. Save some mince, cauli-mash and broccoli for tomorrow's lunch. Make a batch of granola for the week	**Use these tips every day or as often as possible.** ■ Drink a cup of warm water with lemon or apple cider vinegar to start the day. For an extra health kick add turmeric, coconut oil, black pepper or sea salt
■ 2 black coffees a day or 4 cups of black tea* ■ Unlimited water or herbal teas *can add cream to coffee and tea	½ cup kombucha (replace one of your drinks for the day with this) and 30–40g of macadamia nuts	Save some chicken for tomorrow's lunch. Make broth from chicken bones	■ Get 7–9 hours of sleep each night ■ Chew your food slowly ■ Drink water before meals to avoid overeating ■ Take the stairs instead of the lift ■ Eat off smaller plates for portion control
■ 2 black coffees a day or 4 cups of black tea* ■ Unlimited water or herbal teas *can add cream to coffee and tea	1 cup bone broth and 30g of macadamia nuts	Make a batch of seed crackers	■ Get stuck into a good book ■ Set aside some me-time ■ Meditate during your lunch ■ Exercise before work to get energised for the day ■ Spend time in nature ■ Practise 10 minutes of gratitude each day ■ Spend quality time with friends and family
■ 2 black coffees a day or 4 cups of black tea* ■ Unlimited water or herbal teas *can add cream to coffee and tea	1 cup bone broth with 30g fatty biltong	Save some supper for tomorrow's lunch	■ Avoid coffee for a day and see how you feel. Carry on if there's a positive difference ■ Meditate to relax and de-stress before bed ■ Up your exercise game: sprinting, squatting, swimming, skipping, dancing
■ 2 black coffees a day or 4 cups of black tea* ■ Unlimited water or herbal teas *can add cream to coffee and tea	30g of macadamia nuts	Save some fish for tomorrow	■ Reward yourself with a relaxing candle-lit bath ■ Pamper yourself with a foot massage or pedicure ■ Drink a cup of warm water with apple cider vinegar before bed to help lower fasting blood-sugar levels
■ 2 black coffees a day or 4 cups of black tea* ■ Unlimited water or herbal teas *can add cream to coffee and tea	½ cup kombucha (replace one of your drinks with this)	Make sure the sausages you use don't contain gluten. Save some mince etc for tomorrow's lunch. Make extra pancakes for breakfast and store in the fridge	■ Laugh and have fun!
■ 2 black coffees a day or 4 cups of black tea* ■ Unlimited water or herbal teas *can add cream to coffee and tea	Bone broth	Prepare for next week	

4.3 MEAL PLAN: TRANSFORMATION

	BREAKFAST	LUNCH	SUPPER
MONDAY Carbs: 25g Fat: 110–116g Protein: 88–91g	3 fried eggs in butter, 2–3 rashers streaky bacon, ½ grilled tomato, 2 tbsp sauerkraut	½–1 tin tuna in brine with 2–3 tbsp homemade mayo with a salad of 1 cup rocket or other greens, ¼ cucumber, brined pickles, spring onion, drizzled with apple cider vinegar and olive oil/apple vinaigrette with 2 Seed Crackers	Cabhetti Bolognaise: 1 cup mince made with onion, tomato purée/tinned tomatoes, seasoning and green-listed veg on a bed of buttered cabbage
TUESDAY Carbs: 20g Fat: 125g Protein: 94g	2 fillets smoked mackerel with ½ avocado, lemon and 1tbsp cream cheese/soft kefir cheese	Leftover Cabhetti Bolognaise	Chicken Salad with 50g chicken and ½ cup cooked green beans, 1 cup cos lettuce (or other), 1 tbsp Parmesan shavings, 30g bacon bits and 1 boiled egg with homemade mayo and brined pickles
WEDNESDAY Carbs: 24g Fat: 101–111g Protein: 80–101g	2–3 boiled eggs and a smoothie with ½ cup milk kefir, 10 blueberries, 1 tbsp flax seeds, 1 tbsp sunflower seeds	3 buttered Seed Crackers with 1 cup lettuce, brined pickles, 3 slices cheese, 5 cherry tomatoes	100–150g chicken with skin on, 1 cup blanched green beans, ½ cup broccoli with butter and lemon
THURSDAY Carbs: 25–26g Fat: 119–133g Protein: 82–97g	2–3 egg omelette with ½ cup sautéed baby spinach, ½ cup sautéed mushrooms, ¼ cup sautéed onion	3 buttered Seed Crackers with 1 cup lettuce, brined pickles/sauerkraut, 3 slices cheese, 5 cherry tomatoes	100–150g lamb neck chops with Caprese salad, dressed with balsamic vinegar and olive oil
FRIDAY Carbs: 28g Fat:126–137g Protein: 84–92g	2–3 boiled eggs and a smoothie with ½ cup whole-milk kefir, 10 blueberries, 1 tbsp flax seeds, 1 tbsp sunflower seeds	Chicken broth with 100–150g chicken, ½ cup mushrooms and bean sprouts with 2 buttered Seed Crackers	100g rump steak with butter flavoured with garlic and herbs, ½ cup cauliflower with cheese sauce and ½ cup pumpkin
SATURDAY Carbs: 21g Fat: 122–127g Protein: 89–92g	3 fried eggs in butter, 2–3 rashers streaky bacon, ½ grilled tomato, 2 tbsp sauerkraut	Steak salad with 100g leftover steak, 1 cup rocket, ½ avocado, ¼ sliced onion, 5 cherry tomatoes, crumbled feta, sprinkle of sunflower seeds and an apple cider/olive oil dressing with horseradish	Seared salmon fillet on a bed of ½ cup sautéed mushrooms flavoured with ginger and garlic, with ½ cup bok choi, sprinkled with toasted sesame seeds
SUNDAY Carbs: 27g Fat: 115–126g Protein: 91–110g	40g smoked salmon trout with ½ avocado and 2–3 poached eggs with a drizzle of lemon and olive oil	3–4 lamb meatballs, with 2 tbsp homemade tzatziki (yoghurt/kefired sour cream, cucumber, garlic, lemon) ¼ grilled aubergine, and tomato and cucumber salad drizzled with lemon and olive oil	Chicken broth with 100–150g chicken and 1 cup broccoli, 2 buttered Seed Crackers

DRINKS	SNACKS	TIPS	LIFESTYLE TIPS
■ Unlimited water or herbal teas ■ To stay lean, avoid milk in hot drinks	Bone broth (optional if you are still hungry)	Make enough Cabhetti Bolognaise for lunch tomorrow. Make a big batch of chicken bone broth and freeze to use during the week	**Use these tips every day or as often as possible.** ■ Drink a cup of warm water with lemon or apple cider vinegar to start the day. For an extra health kick add turmeric, coconut oil, black pepper or sea salt
■ Unlimited water or herbal teas ■ To stay lean, avoid milk in hot drinks	Bone broth (optional if you are still hungry)	Save some chicken for tomorrow's supper. Make a batch of Seed Crackers for the week	■ Get 7–9 hours of sleep each night ■ Chew your food slowly ■ Drink water before meals to avoid overeating ■ Take the stairs instead of the lift ■ Eat off smaller plates for portion control ■ Get stuck into a good book ■ Set aside some me-time
■ Unlimited water or herbal teas ■ To stay lean, avoid milk in hot drinks	Bone broth (optional if you are still hungry)		■ Meditate during your lunch ■ Exercise before work to get energised for the day ■ Spend time in nature ■ Practise 10 minutes of gratitude each day ■ Spend quality time with friends and family ■ Avoid coffee for a day and see how you feel. Carry on if there's a positive difference
■ Unlimited water or herbal teas ■ To stay lean, avoid milk in hot drinks	Bone broth (optional if you are still hungry)		■ Meditate to relax and de-stress before bed ■ Up your exercise game: sprinting, squatting, swimming, skipping, dancing ■ Reward yourself with a relaxing candle-lit bath
■ Unlimited water or herbal teas ■ To stay lean, avoid milk in hot drinks	Small handful of macadamia nuts (optional if you are still hungry)	Make some extra steak and save for tomorrow's lunch	■ Pamper yourself with a foot massage or pedicure ■ Drink a cup of warm water with apple cider vinegar before bed to help lower fasting blood-sugar levels ■ Laugh and have fun!
■ Unlimited water or herbal teas ■ To stay lean, avoid milk in hot drinks	Bone broth (optional if you are still hungry)		
■ Unlimited water or herbal teas ■ To stay lean, avoid milk in hot drinks	Small handful of macadamia nuts (optional if you are still hungry)	Prepare for next week	

4.3 MEAL PLAN: TRANSFORMATION WITH INTERMITTENT FASTING

	BREAKFAST	LUNCH	SUPPER
MONDAY Carbs: 24–25g Fat: 124–148g Protein: 87–105g	Fast (no food for 16 hours after last night's dinner)	2–3 boiled eggs with 1–2 sausages (beef/pork: no fillers) and salad with a dressing of olive oil and apple cider vinegar/apple vinaigrette	150g rump steak with 1 cup cooked spinach, cauli-mash and 1–2 tbsp simple homemade mushroom sauce (a reduction of cream and mushrooms with seasoning)
TUESDAY Carbs: 27–29g Fat: 122–140g Protein: 91–100g	Drink a cup of warm water with lemon to start the day	150–180g leftover rump steak sliced, with ½–1 avocado, 1 cup rocket, cherry tomatoes, olives, 2 boiled eggs, 1 tbsp sauerkraut, a dressing of olive oil and apple cider vinegar with 2 buttered Seed Crackers	200g grilled/roast chicken (skin on) with ½ cup cooked buttered pumpkin, 1 cup broccoli, ¼ aubergine, and gravy made from pan juices (reduce and add a dollop cold butter)
WEDNESDAY Carbs: 27g Fat: 115–131g Protein: 78–87g	Fast (no food for 16 hours after last night's dinner)	150–180g leftover shredded chicken, 3–4 tbsp homemade mayo, sliced brined pickles, 1 cup watercress, 2–3 buttered seed crackers, sliced cherry tomatoes and ½ avocado	Pork/kassler chop with 1 cup sautéed cabbage, 2 tbsp sauerkraut, ¼ cup sautéed onion, ½ cup cauliflower and 1–2 tbsp simple mustard sauce made with cream and mustard
THURSDAY Carbs: 29–33g Fat: 110–130g Protein: 78–102g	Drink a cup of warm water with lemon to start the day	1–2 leftover pork chops with 1–2 cup sliced cabbage, a handful bean sprouts, 2–3 tbsp homemade mayo, squeeze lemon juice and sprinkled nuts	120–150g grilled fish fillet with lemon butter, ½ cup cauli-mash, 1 cup buttered broccoli and 2 tbsp sauerkraut with a side salad and apple vinaigrette
FRIDAY Carbs: 26–31g Fat:105–119g Protein: 80–89g	Drink a cup of warm water with lemon to start the day	Leftover grilled fish fillet with lemon butter, ½ cup cauli-mash, 1 cup buttered broccoli and 2 tbsp sauerkraut with a side salad and apple vinaigrette	Sliced grilled chicken breast wrapped in lettuce leaves with cucumber slices, mange tout, spring onion, few slices avocado, bean sprouts and fresh herbs with apple vinaigrette and a few sweet potato fries
SATURDAY Carbs: 32–36g Fat: 108–119g Protein: 80–89g	Drink a cup of warm water with lemon to start the day	1–2 burger patties, 1 slice of cheese with cabbage coleslaw and brined pickles	curry with ½ cup cauli-rice and a dollop of yoghurt/kefired sour cream
SUNDAY Carbs: 21–22g Fat: 131–137g Protein: 86–99g	2–3 egg omelette with leftover curry filling and fresh herbs with dollop yoghurt/kefired sour cream		120–150g grilled white fish and a salad of 1 cup roasted pumpkin with ½ cup rocket, 2 tbsp goat's cheese/soft kefir cheese, with sprinkled seeds (pumpkin/ sunflower) and apple vinaigrette

DRINKS	SNACKS	TIPS	LIFESTYLE TIPS
■ Unlimited water or herbal teas ■ To stay lean, avoid milk in hot drinks	Break fast with cup of bone broth	Make extra steak for lunch tomorrow. Make a batch of Seed Crackers. Make a pot of bone broth	**Use these tips every day or as often as possible.**
■ Unlimited water or herbal teas ■ To stay lean, avoid milk in hot drinks	Break fast with cup of bone broth	Keep some chicken for tomorrow's brunch. Make a batch of mayo	■ Drink a cup of warm water with lemon or apple cider vinegar to start the day. For an extra health kick add turmeric, coconut oil, black pepper or sea salt ■ Get 7–9 hours of sleep each night ■ Chew your food slowly ■ Drink water before meals to avoid overeating ■ Take the stairs instead of the lift ■ Eat off smaller plates for portion control
■ Unlimited water or herbal teas ■ To stay lean, avoid milk in hot drinks	Break fast with a handful of nuts	Keep a chop or 2 for tomorrow's lunch	■ Get stuck into a good book ■ Set aside some me-time ■ Meditate during your lunch ■ Exercise before work to get energised for the day ■ Spend time in nature ■ Practise 10 minutes of gratitude each day ■ Spend quality time with friends and family ■ Avoid coffee for a day and see how you feel. Carry on if there's a positive difference
■ Unlimited water or herbal teas ■ To stay lean, avoid milk in hot drinks	Break fast with cup of bone broth	Save some fish for tomorrow's lunch	■ Meditate to relax and de-stress before bed ■ Up your exercise game: sprinting, squatting, swimming, skipping, dancing ■ Reward yourself with a relaxing candle-lit bath
■ Unlimited water or herbal teas ■ To stay lean, avoid milk in hot drinks	Break fast with a handful of macadamia nuts		■ Pamper yourself with a foot massage or pedicure ■ Drink a cup of warm water with apple cider vinegar before bed to help lower fasting blood-sugar levels ■ Laugh and have fun!
■ Unlimited water or herbal teas ■ To stay lean, avoid milk in hot drinks	Break fast with cup of bone broth	Save some curry for tomorrow	
■ Unlimited water or herbal teas ■ To stay lean, avoid milk in hot drinks	Break fast with cup of bone broth	Prepare for next week	

		BREAKFAST	LUNCH	SUPPER
MONDAY Carbs: 43g Fat: 130–141g Protein: 91–107g		Fast (no food for 16 hours after last night's dinner)	Salad of baby spinach, beetroot, avocado, Danish feta and sunflower seeds with 100–120g cooked chicken and a smoothie of kefir, strawberries and almonds	150–200g rump steak with ½ cup broccoli, ½ cup pumpkin and ¼ sweet potato with cheese sauce
TUESDAY Carbs: 52–53g Fat: 121–133g Protein: 94–104g		2–3 fried eggs with grilled tomato, 2–3 rashers bacon, ½ cup wilted spinach	Buttered baked sweet potato with 2 tbsp cream cheese/soft kefir cheese, leftover veg, and leftover rump steak with grated cheese and side salad	1 cup courgette noodles topped with a creamy chicken and mushroom sauce, topped with fresh basil
WEDNESDAY Carbs: 34g Fat: 141g Protein: 87g		Fast (no food for 16 hours after last night's dinner)	Trout and cream cheese/soft kefir cheese omelette with 1 cup watercress, ½ avocado and a smoothie made with ¼ cup coconut milk, ¼ cup yoghurt/kefir, ¼ cup blueberries, ½ tsp xylitol (optional)	Beef mince and caulirice-stuffed peppers, topped with cheese and grilled in the oven with a salad dressed with apple cider vinegar and olive oil
THURSDAY Carbs: 36–51g Fat: 127–162g Protein: 71–88g		Fast (no food for 16 hours after last night's dinner)	Leftover beef mince and caulirice-stuffed peppers topped with cheese and grilled in the oven with an avocado salad dressed with apple cider vinegar and olive oil/apple vinaigrette	Grilled, sliced aubergine topped with homemade tomato sauce, mozzarella and ham/salami, and grilled again to form an open sandwich, with a basic salad and apple vinaigrette
FRIDAY Carbs: 51g Fat:131g Protein: 95g		Fast (no food for 16 hours after last night's dinner)	¼ cup granola (toast a mixture of nuts and seeds with some spices), with 1 cup double-thick yoghurt/kefir, ½ cup strawberries and 2 boiled eggs	Crispy lemon lamb chops with ½ cup buttered pumpkin and 1 cup buttered green beans, sprinkled with flaked almonds
SATURDAY Carbs: 54–58g Fat: 100–133g Protein: 80–97g		Omelette with bacon, spinach and mature cheese (or any green-listed fillings)	Leftover crispy lemon lamb chops with ½ cup buttered pumpkin and 1 cup buttered green beans, sprinkled with flaked almonds with lemon	Classic Chicken Soup for the Soul with chilli, garlic, ginger, 1 cup bok choi and 1 cup broccoli and bean sprouts
SUNDAY Carbs: 57–62g Fat: 124–143g Protein: 87–96g		¼ cup granola (toast a mixture of nuts and seeds with some spices), with 1 cup double-thick yoghur/kefir and a small banana with 1 boiled egg	150–200g grilled white fish with diced roasted sweet potato, diced roasted pumpkin and feta mixed with caulirice to create a salad (1 portion)	Courgette noodles topped with pan-roasted baby tomatoes, basil and cheese

DRINKS	SNACKS	TIPS	LIFESTYLE TIPS
■ 2 cups of coffee or 4 cups of tea ■ Unlimited water or herbal teas ■ ¼–½ cup kombucha	Have some broth or a handful of nuts to break fast if necessary	Make a roast chicken that you can use for lunch on Monday and supper on Tuesday. Make a stock with the bones. Keep some steak and sweet potato for tomorrow	**Use these tips every day or as often as possible.** ■ Drink a cup of warm water with lemon or apple cider vinegar to start the day. For an extra health kick add turmeric, coconut oil, black pepper or sea salt
■ 2 cups of coffee or 4 cups of tea ■ Unlimited water or herbal teas ■ ¼–½ cup kombucha		Use any leftover veggies in the sweet potato	■ Get 7–9 hours of sleep each night ■ Chew your food slowly ■ Drink water before meals to avoid overeating ■ Take the stairs instead of the lift ■ Eat off smaller plates for portion control ■ Get stuck into a good book ■ Set aside some me-time
■ 2 cups of coffee or 4 cups of tea ■ Unlimited water or herbal teas ■ ¼–½ cup kombucha	Have some broth or a handful of nuts to break fast if necessary	Save some supper for lunch tomorrow	■ Meditate during your lunch ■ Exercise before work to get energised for the day ■ Spend time in nature ■ Practise 10 minutes of gratitude each day ■ Spend quality time with friends and family
■ 2 cups of coffee or 4 cups of tea ■ Unlimited water or herbal teas ■ ¼–½ cup kombucha			■ Avoid coffee for a day and see how you feel. Carry on if there's a positive difference ■ Meditate to relax and de-stress before bed ■ Up your exercise game: sprinting, squatting, swimming, skipping, dancing ■ Reward yourself with a relaxing candle-lit bath
■ 2 cups of coffee or 4 cups of tea ■ Unlimited water or herbal teas ■ ¼–½ cup kombucha	A handful of fatty biltong	Save some supper for tomorrow's lunch. Make a batch of granola	■ Pamper yourself with a foot massage or pedicure ■ Drink a cup of warm water with apple cider vinegar before bed to help lower fasting blood-sugar levels ■ Laugh and have fun!
■ 2 cups of coffee or 4 cups of tea ■ Unlimited water or herbal teas ■ ¼–½ cup kombucha			
■ 2 cups of coffee or 4 cups of tea ■ Unlimited water or herbal teas ■ ¼–½ cup kombucha		Prepare for next week	

GLOSSARY-INDEX

Adrenaline: the "fight or flight" hormone; usually released in response to danger; it prepares the body for imminent action by, among other things, raising blood-sugar and thus insulin levels. For a full list of hormones that affect the diet see p53. For more on what adrenaline influences read *The Pie of Life* from p50.

Alcohol: it's a grey area. See p152.

Appestat: the region in the hypothalamus of the brain that is believed to control a person's appetite for food. See a full explanation on p51-2 and *The Science* from p28.

Cholesterol: a compound made by the body which, among other functions, is essential to give cell walls their strength and suppleness. Controversially demonised by the diet-heart hypothesis. For a fuller explanation see *What about my cholesterol?* on p165-6. Also see p31, 33 and 168.

Chronic disease: long-lasting diseases and disorders, such as type-2 diabetes and high blood pressure, which tend to be managed but never cured; as opposed to acute diseases and disorders which are short-term. For a summary of the chronic diseases and disorders associated with the modern carb-heavy diet, see *From Icebergs To Volcanoes* on p45.

Chronic inflammation: long-term inflammation. See *The Four Horsemen Of The Carb-pocalypse* from p36, in general; and p42-3, in particular.

Coeliac disease: a type of hypersensitivity to gluten. See p41. Compare *Non-coeliac gluten sensitivity*.

Coronary heart disease: plaque build-up inside the coronary arteries (often just "heart disease"). See *What about my cholesterol?* on p165-6; also see p32, 34 and 47.

Cortisol: the "stress hormone"; released in response to stress, it raises blood-sugar and thus insulin levels. For a full list of hormones that affect the diet see p53. For more on what cortisol influences read section *The Pie of Life* from p50.

Dairy: usually great, sometimes problematic. See p147.

Endorphins: uplifting hormones that depress pain and increase feelings of wellbeing. For a full list of hormones that affect the diet see p53. For more on what endorphins influence read section *The Pie of Life* from p50.

Fatty acids: a basic storage unit of energy for the body; can be saturated, unsaturated or polyunsaturated. Trans fats are fatty acids not found in natural foods but arise from the manufacture of vegetable oils; they are associated with increased risk of coronary heart disease. See *How is a ketogenic diet related to the RMR diet?* on p164 and *What about my cholesterol?* on p165-6.

Fertilisers: any foods and drinks that help restore the health of the gut, whether the gut lining or the gut microbiota (gut flora). Fermented foods, broths and natural probiotics are all fertilisers. See *Fertilise your gut* on p115; *Restoration station* from p190; and the recipes that follow.

Glucose: simple sugars broken down from dietary carbohydrates used for energy; raises insulin levels. See p24; *Insulin resistance* on p37-8; *Restoration* on p110; *How is a ketogenic diet related to the RMR diet?* on p164; and *Your Insulin Resistance And General Health* on p167-8. Compare *Ketone bodies*.

Gluten: a component of wheat and other grains now believed to cause havoc on the body's immune system and general health. See *Gluten sensitivity* on p40-2, in particular; and *The Four Horsemen Of The Carbpocalypse* from p36, in general.

Insulin: the fat-building hormone. For a full list of hormones that affect the diet see p53. For more on what insulin influences read section *The Pie of Life* from p50. See *Insulin resistance*.

Insulin resistance: a failure of the body to respond as it should when insulin is secreted, resulting in ever-increasing levels of insulin, leading eventually to type-2 diabetes and other health complications. For a full explanation and more on why this is important see p16. Also see *What is insulin resistance and why are hormones so important?* on p24-5; *The Four Horsemen Of The Carb-pocalypse* from p36, in general, and p37-8 in particular; and *Your Insulin Resistance And General Health* on p167-8.

Irritable bowel syndrome (IBS): recurring abdominal pain, diarrhoea or constipation. See *Gut problems* on p38-40 and *Gluten sensitivity* on p40-2.

Ketone bodies: bodies produced by the liver from fatty acids used for energy, generally after glycogen stores (which store glucose) have been depleted. See p110 and *How is a ketogenic diet related to the RMR diet?* on p164. See *Ketosis*. Compare *Glucose*.

Ketosis: The metabolic state in which the body derives its energy largely from ketone bodies; a natural state when consuming a very low-carb healthy-fat (ketogenic) diet. See p110 and *How is a ketogenic diet related to the RMR diet?* on p164.

Leaky gut syndrome: syndrome in which the tight junctions between the cells in the gut lining separate and the content of the small intestine enters the bloodstream. See *The Four Horsemen of the Carb-pocalypse* from p36, in general; *Gluten sensitivity* on p40-2; and *Chronic inflammation* on p42-3.

Leptin: the satiety hormone; decreases appetite. For a full list of hormones that affect the diet see p53. For more on what leptin influences read section *The Pie of Life* from p50.

Metabolic syndrome: a group of risk factors, including increased blood pressure, high blood sugar, excess fat around the waist and abnormal cholesterol or triglyceride levels, that raise the risk of heart disease, stroke, diabetes and other health problems. For more on how metabolic syndrome is affected by carbohydrates, see *The Four Horsemen Of The Carb-pocalypse* from p36. For a fuller list, see *From Icebergs To Volcanoes* from p45.

Nightshades: plants of the *Solanaceae* family that include tomatoes, potatoes, peppers and aubergines; believed to be problematic to some. See *The "deadly" nightshades* on p151.

Non-coeliac gluten sensitivity: a type of hypersensitivity to gluten. See p42. Compare *Coeliac disease*.

Probiotics: the pharmaceutical equivalent of naturally fermented foods. See *Fermented foods v probiotics* on p116 and *Probiotic-rich foods* on p207-8.

Pregnancy: see *Who should not fast?* on p138 and *Can I eat this way if I'm pregnant?* on p162.

Recipes: for the full list of basic RMR diet and restorative recipes in this book see p185; for mostly Restoration-appropriate recipes see *Real Meal Revolution: Raising Superheroes*; for mostly Transformation-appropriate recipes see *The Real Meal Revolution*.

Saturated fats: animal and coconut fat products, unfairly maligned by the diet-heart hypothesis and subsequent dietary guidelines. See p34.

Supplements: vitamins, minerals and nutrients taken to rectify dietary deficiencies; Real Meal Revolution distinguishes between bottled/ bought supplements and real-food supplements, encouraging the latter wherever possible. See *Restoration station* on p190-2 and the recipes that follow.

Thyroid hormones: hormones that regulate metabolism, among other things. For a full list of hormones that affect the diet see p53. For more on what thyroid hormones influence read section *The Pie of Life* from p50.

Visceral fat: the body fat around the belly, the presence of which is a likely indicator of insulin resistance; considered more harmful than fat found under the skin. See p100.

Zonulin: a protein that modulates the permeability of tight junctions between cells of the wall of the digestive tract; can be affected by gluten to cause leaky gut syndrome. See *Gluten sensitivity* on p40-2.

ACKNOWLEDGEMENTS

Before I get to the people who were involved in the creation of this book, a special mention goes to my wife Kate and daughter Imogen. Thank you for being in my corner through each round of entrepreneurial beatings and victories, lessons and epiphanies.

This is a list of key people who dedicated time and energy into filtering the information in this book from the all-consuming information created by the Real Meal Revolution tsunami. Without the blood, sweat and tears of each of these Superheroes, *Real Meal 2.0* may have only ended up at Real Meal 1.5. I honestly believe the world is a better place as a result of the writing, designing, fact-checking, analysing, arguing, rewriting, coding, charting, stressing, debating, discussing and rehashing that each of you put into this project.

First up, special thanks to Leaine Brebner, our Content Queen, who put so much thought and care into the groundwork behind this book. And to Steve, Penny, Rob, Agent Smith, Matt, Stehan, The Flaxinator, Kathy, Monty and Muffin at the Real Meal Revolution – you are legends.

Then, to the best book team in the world:

Tim Richman – The Tarantino

Liz Sarant – The Whip

Simon Richardson – The Warhol

Bridget Surtees – The White Knight

Karen Hartzenberg – The Referee

Guss Davey – The Zuckerberg

Jody Doyle – The Harvey Specter of Banting

Dr Ian Proudfoot – The Enforcer, moral compass and my dad

And, of course, a big thank you to the experts. We've listed key figures in our Real Meal journey in *The Experts* section, but we're indebted to all the doctors, scientists, nutritionists, coaches, psychologists and general legends whose work we devour and digest to bring to our clients and readers the very best we can to help change lives. Your wisdom and courage allows us the opportunity to help people on a daily basis; without you at the coal face, we'd have nothing to power us, fat or otherwise. In particular, thank you to my good friend and personal expert, the one and only Prof Tim Noakes.

Jonno Proudfoot

TO LEARN ABOUT BECOMING A
REAL MEAL REVOLUTION CERTIFIED COACH
(OR ANYTHING ELSE IN THIS BOOK),
SEE WWW.REALMEALREVOLUTION.COM.

FOR THE COMPLETE REAL LISTS, TURN THE PAGE

FOR THE COMPLETE REAL LISTS, TURN THE PAGE

GREEN EAT TO HUNGER

(p) – 'prebiotic' or 'high fibre'
(e) – high in digestive enzymes
(n) – Night Shades (see p151)

THE COMPLETE REAL LISTS

FRUIT & VEGETABLES
- All green leafy vegetables
- Artichoke hearts (p)
- Asparagus (p)
- Aubergine (n)
- Avocado (p)
- Bean sprouts
- Beans such as green, runner, broad (p)
- Broccoli (p)
- Brussels sprouts (p)
- Cabbage (p)
- Cauliflower (p)
- Celery (p)
- Chard (p)
- Courgettes
- Cucumber
- Endive (p)
- Fennel (p)
- Garlic (p)
- Gem squash
- Kale (p)
- Leeks (p)
- Lemons & limes
- Lettuce
- Mange tout (p)
- Mushrooms
- Onions (p)
- Okra
- Palm hearts (p)
- Peppers (all kinds) (n)
- Radicchio (p)
- Radishes (p)
- Rhubarb
- Rocket (p)
- Shallots (p)
- Spinach (p)
- Spring onions
- Tomatoes (n)
- Turnips
- Watercress (p)

DRINKS
- Caffeine-free herbal teas (with real slices of fruit and herbs)
- Flavoured waters from RMR recipes or other recipes that follow the lists
- Water – sparkling or still

PROTEINS
Free-range, organic and as natural as possible
- All meats, poultry and game
- All naturally cured meats like pancetta, parma ham, coppa, bacon, salami, biltong, jerky
- All offal (highly recommended)
- All seafood
- Eggs

CONDIMENTS
- All vinegars, flavourings and condiments are okay provided they are without sugar, gluten, preservatives or vegetable oils
- Tamari/fermented soy sauce

FERTILISERS
- All homemade bone broths
- Coconut yoghurt
- Coconut kefir
- Kefir butter/cheese
- Kimchi
- Milk kefir
- Naturally fermented pickles
- Sauerkraut

FATS
- Any rendered animal fat (lard, tallow, duck and bacon fat)
- Avocado oil (cold-pressed is best) (e)
- Butter or ghee
- Coconut oil (e)
- Firm cheeses like cheddar, emmental and gouda
- Hard cheeses like parmesan and pecorino
- Macadamia oil (e)
- Mayonnaise, free from preservatives and seed oil
- Nut oils like groundnut oil (as long as they're not heated during extraction or cooking)
- Olive oil (extra virgin) (e)
- Seeds (p)

ORANGE EXERCISE SELF-CONTROL

NUTS

Closed handful (2 tbsp)
- All raw nuts (p)
- Homemade or unprocessed sugar-free nut butters

DAIRY

Unpasteurised is better (¼ cup)
- Cottage cheese, cream, cream cheese, full-fat yoghurt (homemade first, commercial second), sour cream/crème fraîche
- Full-fat cheeses like brie, camembert, gorgonzola, roquefort
- Milk
- Milk substitutes: almond milk, rice milk, coconut milk and hemp milk
- Soft cheeses like mozzarella, feta, ricotta

FRUIT & VEGETABLES

No more than half a closed handful
- Beetroot and golden beets
- Berries – blackberries, blueberries, gooseberries, raspberries, strawberries
- Butternut squash
- Calabash
- Carrots (p)
- Casava
- Celeriac
- Corn on the cob, baby corn
- Hubbard squash
- Jicama
- Papaya (e)
- Parsnips
- Peas (mange tout, garden peas and sugar-snaps) (p)
- Pineapple (e)
- Plantain
- Pumpkin
- Rutabagas
- Spaghetti squash (p)
- Sweet potatoes (p)
- Taro

DRINKS
- Tea (caffeinated)
- Coffee

LEGUMES/ PULSES
- All legumes (best prepared soaked before cooked or sprouted)
- Alfalfa (sprouts) (p)
- Cannellini, kidney and black-eyed (fresh or dried)
- Chickpeas (sprouted or dried)
- Lentils (sprouted or dried)
- Peanuts (raw or in shells only)

FERTILISERS
- Water kefir
- Kombucha

FRUITS & VEGETABLES
- Apples (p)
- Apricots
- Bananas
- Breadfruit
- Cherries
- Edamame
- Figs (only fresh)
- Granadillas
- Grapes
- Guavas
- Jackfruit
- Kiwi fruit
- Kumquats
- Litchis
- Loquats
- Mangoes
- Oranges, clementines and tangerines
- Peaches and nectarines
- Pears and prickly pears
- Persimmon
- Plums
- Pomegranates
- Potatoes (n)
- Quinces
- Starfruit
- Tamarind pulp
- Watermelon

LIGHT RED HARDLY EVER

(p) – 'prebiotic' or 'high fibre'
(e) – high in digestive enzymes
(n) – Night Shades (see p151)

VEGETABLE JUICES/ SMOOTHIES
- Fruit or yoghurt smoothies without frozen yoghurt or ice cream
- Vegetable juices with no added fruit juice

TREATS AND CHOCOLATE
- Dark chocolate (80% and above)
- Dried fruit
- Honey
- Pure maple syrup

GLUTEN-FREE GRAINS AND GRAIN PRODUCTS
- Amaranth
- Arrowroot
- Buckwheat
- Bran
- Gluten-free pasta
- Millet
- Oats (must be gluten-free)
- Popcorn
- Quinoa
- Rices – whole grain, arborio, sushi, jasmine, Thai and rice noodles
- Sorghum
- Tapioca
- Teff

FLOURS
Non-GMO and gluten-free should be a standard rule
- Almond flour
- Coconut flour
- Corn flour
- Chickpea flour
- Maize meal
- Pea flour
- Polenta
- Rice flour

GREY IT'S A GREY AREA

THE COMPLETE REAL LISTS

TREATS
- LCHF baked goods, including cakes, cupcakes or any sugar-free desserts
- Sugar-free ice cream

SWEETENERS
- Erythritol
- Isomalt
- Stevia powder
- Sucralose
- Xylitol

DRINKS
- All alcoholic beverages
- Protein shakes
- Supplements

VEGETARIAN PROTEINS
- Naturally fermented tofu
- Pea protein
- Processed soy

REALLY RED NEVER EVER

GENERAL
- Any food with added sugar
- Crisps
- Fast food (unless you trust the brand and you know the ingredients)
- Sugary condiments like ketchup, marinades and salad dressings, unless they are free from sugar and other nasties

SWEET THINGS
- All confectionery and (non-dark) chocolates (including 'protein', 'energy' or 'breakfast'/'snack' bars)
- Artificial sweeteners – aspartame, acesulfame K, saccharin
- Agave
- Canned fruit
- Coconut blossom sugar
- Cordials
- Fructose
- Glucose
- Jam
- Malt
- Rice malt syrup
- Sugar – white, caster, icing, light brown, dark brown
- Sugar-cured or commercially pickled foods
- Golden syrup

FOODS CONTAINING GLUTEN
- All flours and all breads made from grains containing gluten
- Barley
- Bulgur
- Couscous
- Durum
- Einkorn
- Farina
- Graham flour
- Kamut
- Matzo
- Orzo
- Rye
- Semolina
- Spelt
- Triticale
- Wheat
- Wheat germ

OTHER GRAIN-BASED PRODUCTS
- All commercial breaded or battered foods (breaded chicken nuggets, battered fish, etc)
- All commercial breakfast cereals (muesli, granola, corn flakes, coco pops, cold porridges, etc)
- All crackers and cracker breads

DRINKS
- All energy drinks
- All soft drinks, including diet drinks
- Commercial fruit juices
- Commercial iced teas
- Flavoured milk and milkshakes

DAIRY-RELATED
- Commercial cheese spreads
- Coffee creamers
- Condensed milk
- Ice cream and commercial frozen yoghurt

FATS
- All industrial seed and vegetable oil derivatives
- Butter spreads
- Canola oil
- Cottonseed oil
- Corn oil
- Margarine and shortening
- Rice bran oil
- Sunflower oil
- Safflower oil

PROTEINS
- Highly processed sausages and luncheon meats
- Meats cured with excessive sugar

"I have type-1 diabetes, and I was on a low-fat low-GI diet for more than 25 years. I was taught that with having diabetes I should not eat fats, and that I should rather eat low-GI carbs, to keep my blood sugar stable. I then decided to do extensive research on the LCHF lifestyle. This lifestyle seemed perfect for me, and I was hooked! Since I began the RMR diet, I have lost a stone, and I have reduced my short act insulin by two-thirds."

– NINA, 53

"I cured my hepatitis C genotype 5 with LCHF and lost eight dress sizes. I will never eat any other way."
– ANYA, 58

"After starting the RMR diet I ran my best ever Comrades marathon and I have managed to maintain my weight loss over the past three years."
– HEATHER, 47

★ ★ ★ ★ ★

"I am an avid endurance athlete, and compete in Iron Man distance triathlons. After turning 40 it seemed harder to keep healthy and injury-free during the training I needed to put in. The RMR diet helped me reduce inflammation, provide a steady source of energy and, importantly, keep me lean. I haven't been injured or even had a cold since I started."
– DAVID, 41